Nursing the
Psychiatric Patient

Nursing the Psychiatric Patient

Joan Burr
R.M.N., S.R.N.

*King's Fund Administrative Course; formerly Deputy
Matron, the Bethlem Royal and the Maudsley Hospitals, London,
and Deputy Principal of the King's Fund Staff College
for Ward Sisters*

and

Una V. Budge
R.M.N., S.R.N., R.N.T.

*Senior Nursing Officer (Education),
Tooting Bec Hospital, London, and
Examiner for the General Nursing
Council for England and Wales
and for Northern Ireland*

Third Edition

**Baillière Tindall
London**

A BAILLIÈRE TINDALL book published by
Cassell Ltd
35 Red Lion Square, London WC1R 4SG
and at Sydney, Auckland, Toronto, Johannesburg,
an affiliate of
Macmillan Publishing Co., Inc.,
New York

© 1976 Baillière Tindall
a division of Cassell Ltd

First published 1967
Second edition 1970
Reprinted 1974
Third edition 1976
Reprinted 1979

ISBN 0 7020 0614 9

Printed in Great Britain by
Lowe & Brydone Printers Limited, Thetford, Norfolk

Contents

Preface

During the last few years there have been fundamental changes in the administration of local authorities and psychiatric hospitals and in the career structure of trained nurses. Lines of communication and responsibility have been changed; some posts have become obsolete and new ones have been created, while a whole new system of job titles has appeared. These changes have had a radical effect on the work of hospital administrators, medical staff and senior nursing staff and to a lesser extent on the work of all trained nursing staff.

But this book is not intended for trained nurses. It is written for pupil nurses and for student nurses in the early part of their training. Here the need is still for the nurse to learn the meaning of a therapeutic nurse–patient relationship and to develop her skills in this field.

The most important changes that have taken place in the nursing of psychiatric patients over the last ten years are those which have been brought about by changes in attitudes towards mental illness. There is a more relaxed atmosphere in the wards of psychiatric hospitals. Staff no longer feel that they must be authoritarian or over-protective. Routine is less rigid, patients have more opportunity to question and criticize and there are fewer rules. Nurses are more aware of the patient's psychological needs as a person. They have learned to see the sick individual as someone's mother, brother, daughter or employee with a place in the world, uniquely his own, instead of a 'case' of depression or schizophrenia.

This book is about attitudes. It sets out to help the newcomer in psychiatric nursing to see Mrs Brown or Tom Jones as a person and to rescue and maintain those areas in which the sick person is still whole and normal. Without such understanding and awareness on the part of nurses, any treatment becomes less effective and may even be useless.

In preparing this revised edition I have had the valuable help of Miss Una Budge, R.M.N., S.R.N., R.N.T., Senior Nursing Officer (Education), Tooting Bec Hospital, London. I would like to say how grateful I am for her assistance.

Many changes in job descriptions and job titles have, of course, been necessary. We have also taken out the chapter on patients with epilepsy because, owing to improved medication, epileptic fits are rarely seen in hospitals now and these patients' need for hospital treatment arises from the fact that they have developed some psychiatric problem, probably as a result of the social difficulties which they face as epileptics. In the place of this chapter we have included a chapter on patients with organic disorders among which epilepsy is included. Epilepsy, in itself, is no longer regarded as a mental illness and a description of an epileptic fit would perhaps nowadays more properly be found in a textbook on First Aid.

Added emphasis has been given to the need for developing the nurses' skill in helping institutionalized patients; the descriptions of some physical treatments have been shortened, as these are not widely used now; the chapter on drugs has been up-dated, and the growing need for better provision by local authorities for discharged patients has been stressed, including the urgent need to give support to the relatives of these patients.

Preface

This book is not a text book. It is not even about psychiatric nursing in the technical sense. It is about the fundamental attitudes which all nurses must develop if they are to be successful in nursing the mentally ill. I hope that they will enjoy reading it and that it will help and encourage them at the beginning of their training in this fascinating profession.

Marple, Cheshire   JOAN BURR
January 1976

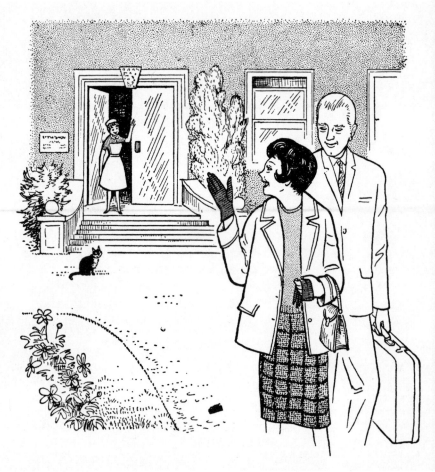

Seventy per cent of the people admitted for mental illness go home again in less than three months, and many within six weeks

1

Human development

A newborn baby wants just two things—love and food. He only knows one way of getting them and that is by yelling. So he yells and along comes milk, softness, warmth, support and lovely reassuring murmurs all around him.

'You know you're a little tyrant!' says his mother as she cuddles him close—and so he is. He is king of a wonderful world in which all his dreams come true.

At first he doesn't know how this happens because he is not aware of his mother as a separate person. He and the food and the love are all part of one safe, enfolding whole. But gradually he begins to tell the difference. He becomes aware of the arm that cradles him so safely. He begins to know that when he is hungry it is his mother who brings food, when he is cold she brings warmth and when he is in pain she picks him up and the pain goes. By himself he is completely helpless, so all his longing for love and food is centred on her, but this blissful state of affairs soon changes. He finds there are times when he cries and no food comes. The wonderful mother who can meet all his needs sometimes refuses to do so and he hates her for it.

Here is emotional conflict right at the beginning of the child's life.

At first his response is violent anger. Look at a scream-ing baby, the contorted face, the clenched fists and kick-

3

ing legs and imagine what would happen if he had the physical strength to match his rage. But as he grows he learns that although he may sometimes have to wait his needs will be met in time. He begins to tolerate frustration and change and this is a very important step in his development.

Right from the beginning of life we all want to get out of unpleasant situations and into pleasant ones. We all have to come to terms with the fact that we cannot always get what we want immediately.

The baby grows into infancy and his simple love-hate response to his mother begins to develop into feelings of delight, pleasure and affection when things go well, or fear, distress, anger and jealousy when he is thwarted. At the same time he is developing physically, beginning to walk, speaking his first words, learning to feed himself and to control his bladder and bowels. All these activities are immensely satisfying to a child. He is endlessly curious about his own body and what it will do, about other people and about anything he can get his hands on. He loves to touch his body. Being cuddled and fondled is a delight to him. His newly discovered skills fascinate him and he expects his mother to be just as pleased if he presents her with a bowel motion as she is if he repeats a new word correctly.

His mother's attitude at this time can affect his emotional development profoundly. He must learn how to behave in a way that is acceptable to other people, but if he is not allowed to feel the pleasure of these early discoveries and achievements he may be unable to grow easily into the next phase.

He may, in effect, remain a child in some ways all his life, or he may return to childish ways of behaving when he is under stress in later life. This return is called regression.

His mother will show approval at certain behaviour and disapproval or anger at other behaviour. This will be distressing or even frightening to the child who now has to control some of his new activities, which to him are so enjoyable, in order to please the mother he loves. He is learning to give up something he wants for fear of losing the approval he wants even more, and in the process he both loves and hates his mother.

As he grows older he will try to please her by doing as she wishes, by becoming like her, even by copying the way she speaks and behaves, like the little boy who bounced into his seat in the bus and said in a weary voice, 'It's nice to take the weight off your feet, isn't it?'

If his mother is tolerant, patient and warm in her attitude he will feel secure in her affection and will come to understand that it is possible for her to be angry with him at times and yet to go on loving him. This helps him to accept his own love-hate feelings towards her and later towards other people.

Fantasy plays a big part in his life at this time. Many children make believe they have a playmate who goes with them everywhere. In their imagination they do many things which they then recount as if they had really happened. Sometimes a child will project his own bad behaviour on to a toy. 'Teddy didn't eat his dinner.' 'It was Teddy making a noise.'

The whole of his life at this stage is a battlefield between his own impulses and the demands of the outside world. Gradually he learns what is acceptable. It is a painful process and he often takes one step back for every two forwards. In an effort to avoid unhappiness he pushes some of his feelings out of his mind altogether, such as his wish to hurt his mother, his fear that she may stop loving him, or his enjoyment of the way his body works. He forgets them so completely that it is as if he had never felt them.

This forgetting is called repression and it is a normal part of growing up at this age, but if too much is re-

5

pressed the child does not learn to cope with his own feelings and these repressed conflicts may result in emotional difficulties in adult life. If he knows that his mother loves him and wants him in spite of everything he becomes able to put up with temporary frustrations and comes to terms with the conventions of ordinary society.

So far his attention has been fixed on his mother, but by about four years old a little boy becomes more aware of his father. At this age he is often rebellious and although he loves and admires his father he regards him also as a figure of authority. 'You wait till your father comes home!' says his exasperated mother. So admiration mingles with fear of punishment.

He also begins to feel jealous of the affection his father gets from his mother. A little boy will run and clutch at his mother when she is doing something for his father, trying to get her attention for himself. He feels guilty over his jealousy and tries to make things right by becoming like his father, doing as he does, saying what he says. He identifies with him and everything has to be 'like Daddy's'.

A little girl, on the other hand, is often very affectionate towards her father, running to meet him, sitting on his knee and gazing up at him with adoring eyes. She begins to look on her mother as a rival for his attention. Like the boy, she finds herself in a conflict of love and jealousy. She tries to make up for it by identifying with her mother. She copies her in every way she can, loves to try on her shoes and hats and picks up turns of phrase that her mother uses. 'Hallo', says a four-year-old, 'It's not bad today, is it?'

So the stage is set in childhood for us to try out relationships with others, not only with our parents, but with brothers and sisters, grandparents and other relatives. The way in which we develop at this time determines to a large extent how we shall react as adults to other men and women. Friendship, love and marriage may all be affected by our early experience of relationships within the family circle.

Going to school is the next big landmark. This may be the first time a child has been separated from his mother and his attitude will depend on how much independence his mother has helped him to reach so far. At school his teachers will give him some of the affection and security he has until now received entirely from his parents. He must learn not only how to read and write but how to mix with other children and to obey new rules without constantly running back to his mother. Some of his affection and hostility towards his parents will now be transferred to his teacher.

A whole new world opens up for him, often one which because of its widened horizons he feels unable to communicate. 'What did you do at school today, Jimmy?' 'Oh, nothing!' he says with a shrug.

This is the time for wearing uniforms, joining clubs, collecting badges, knowing the right passwords and catchphrases. Sport becomes important. His hero might be an Olympic champion and so he goes in for training in a big way. His own demands upon himself are high at this time. He longs to do well, to beat the others, to be accepted and applauded in his own set.

Gradually he is drawing away from the total absorption in his parents. He becomes aware of them as two people in their own right. When he was younger it was their love for him which concerned him so much. Now their relationship to each other becomes equally important for him. He doesn't want them to be over-demonstrative but he does need to feel quite certain that they love each other. His security at this stage depends so much on this certainty that any disharmony between them can have a lasting effect on him. Quarrels, angry

7

arguments or a bitter silence can cause great heartache and bewilderment.

If at this time his parents also demand the maximum effort from him, if he must be first in everything and top of every class, the accumulative effect may be too much. His progress in school work may suffer and his own developing relationships with other people may become unsure. He may try to escape by playing his teacher off against his parents. Instead of moving outwards to meet the world he may turn in on himself, retreating into a world of make-believe where, once again, he has only to wish and it will all come true. Regression to bedwetting and temper tantrums is not uncommon at nine or ten, but for most children this is a time of rapid development physically, mentally and emotionally. A time when, given the security of a stable and affectionate home, they will advance rapidly to the next stage of adolescence.

ADOLESCENCE

During adolescence some young people develop very quickly. Others are slow starters and seem to be children still for a time. Some go through this stage relatively smoothly, others are full of turbulence and crisis.

Physically there are great changes taking place. The boy's voice has deepened and he starts to shave. The girl's figure takes on the curves of a woman. Both have an increased growth of bodily hair. The boy experiences seminal emissions and the girl starts to menstruate.

Along with this physical growth comes a greatly increased sexuality. Each feels an intense interest in the opposite sex. If early questions about sex have been answered truthfully they may be able to handle this increased sexual energy without too much stress, but if sex education has been inadequate there may be much distress and worry. Under the disguise of sophistication there may be much misunderstanding. 'Masturbation

8

will make you insane.' 'People can tell by your face if you've had sex.' 'Kissing can give you a baby.' 'To feel attracted to one of your own sex is the unforgivable sin.' And so the old wives' tales go on. Often a flippant, couldn't-care-less attitude hides ignorance and unhappiness.

The need for support and guidance continues, but now there is an equally strong need to break away from the family, to rebel against the parents' authority. A few are so disturbed that they must hit back in cruelty and destruction, finding a spurious support in the gang, but the majority find help in youth clubs, social groups, sports associations and other leisure-time activities. Here they may meet adults more experienced than themselves, to whom they can talk perhaps with greater ease than to their parents.

Transitory homosexual relationships are normal at this stage. The intense loyalty felt by young people for those in their own group can lead to attachments with someone of the same age. Attachments to older people of the same sex may develop through a need for someone to fill the place of the parent, against whom the young person is rebelling. Gradually the group begins to take an interest in the opposite sex, although the first members to do so may be regarded as disloyal by the others, or teased as cissies.

Most young people are intensely idealistic and deeply serious discussions on religion, love and politics take place at this age. Many of them find meaning and purpose in voluntary work for old or disabled people, or with organized charities.

As they approach maturity their relationships become more settled, until in their turn they begin to look towards marriage and parenthood. How they respond to the challenge of earning a living, choosing a mate and bringing up their own children will depend very much on the patterns of behaviour built into them by their parents.

What a child needs most is steady affection. The two extremes of rejection, or smothering possessive love are both inimical to natural growth, but a warm acceptance in his own family will give him the emotional security to find his own way to adulthood.

ADULT LIFE

As adult men and women we find that we have certain needs which must be met at least partially if we are to lead a full and satisfying life. These are to earn a living, to find love and companionship with the opposite sex, to get on well with other people and to enjoy our leisure.

WORK

Most of us have to earn our own living. We work in order to get money to buy the things we want—food, clothes, a house and furniture, books, music, flowers and all the possessions we love to have around us.

This can mean working long and sometimes irregular hours, getting up at a set time whether we want to or not, taking a training, obeying rules and being corrected when we break them, accepting the authority of senior people often without the opportunity to question, perhaps carrying out monotonous duties which have little meaning for us.

A lot of this happened to us as children when we had to obey our parents and learn the rules of acceptable behaviour. Now it happens in the adult world and again we find ourselves wanting something and having to put up with certain frustrations in order to get it.

The way we behaved as children will affect what we do now. The pattern of behaviour is already set. Some people are always getting on the wrong side of the boss. They feel that they are being victimized, that their true worth is not appreciated. Angry and disillusioned they move from job to job always looking for the right one. Each time they say it will be different, and indeed everything goes well for a time. Then the old trouble starts again. Their friends notice that although each boss is different the arguments are always the same. Instead of 'boss' read 'parents' and we can see that these people are still rebelling against the mother or father, or the teacher, with whom they couldn't come to terms as children.

Others find work an anxiety because they cannot accept responsibility, are afraid to make a decision on their own in case it should be the wrong one. Doubting themselves and their own abilities they need constantly to be told they are doing well, and the slightest criticism plunges them into despair. In their hearts they are still trying to please Mum and Dad, uncertain whether what they do will bring a caress or a slap, guilty when they fail and wanting always the approval and love they were never quite sure they deserved.

Others again drive themselves to extremes. They must get promotion, beat the next man, get a bigger rise, buy a bigger car. The boss has only to suggest that the job is difficult for them to insist that they can take it on—and more. Perhaps without knowing it they are still fighting to keep up with that older brother or sister who was always one step ahead, or still trying so hard to please the parents who always expected them to be top of the class.

Yet work suited to our ability and successfully carried out can be a source of the greatest satisfaction to all of us. Through our work we make a contribution to the good of society, we provide for ourselves and those dependent on us, we come to feel we have value. We realize a sense of achievement that comes from striving with others towards a common goal.

SEX

One of our strongest impulses is to find a mate and have children. Some people find most of their difficulties in this area of life because it is in our sexual relationships more than in any other that the patterns learnt in childhood have their effect. We think we have found the ideal partner only to discover later on that he or she has changed and is not the person we thought. Has he really changed, or did we want an imaginary person rather than a real partner.

Some of us are still looking for our ideal parents when we marry. The young man is attracted to a woman twice his age. Unconsciously he seeks in her the mother who will give him all her love and attention, secure in the thought that this time there is no rival father figure in the background. The girl finds an older man so much more understanding than the boys of her own age. Unconsciously she is still under her father's spell. None of her boy friends comes up to the idealized picture she has of him, and when an older man comes along she sinks back with relief into the childhood relationship of adoring young daughter with experienced and devoted father.

Some who found in childhood that all relationships brought pain, go through life turning from one superficial partnership to another. Afraid to make a deep relationship with another person they try to get the emotional satisfaction they need from a series of temporary liaisons. Others, brought up to repress the pleasure they felt in their own bodies, now feel guilty about their sexual pleasure, and what could have been a delight becomes a furtive indulgence or a frigid duty.

Most people reach adult life capable of making a realistic choice of partner and achieve sufficient maturity to enter into a deep and lasting relationship, but for some the adjustment is too great and sexual relationships bring

12

them a certain amount of difficulty throughout their lives.

SOCIAL RELATIONSHIPS

Psychologists sometimes divide people into two large groups, the extroverts and the introverts.

An extrovert is someone who loves to be with other people. He joins clubs, goes about with a gang of friends and jumps at any excuse to have a party. Faced with a problem he would rather do something active than sit down and think it out. He is curious about what other people are doing and saying. When he is happy he carries others along with his good spirits and when he is depressed everyone knows about it. Physically he is often short, with a round body and a round head on a short neck.

The introvert prefers his own society to that of other people. He would rather go for a walk by himself than to a dance. His hobbies tend to be of a solitary kind and he is more likely to be seen fishing than racing up and down a football field. He enjoys reading and study. Emotionally he does not go up and down on a switchback like the extrovert but has a much more even temperament. When he is happy he is enthusiastic about his intellectual pursuits and if he gets depressed he tends to withdraw into himself, spending much time in daydreaming. Physically he is often tall and angular with a narrow head and slender hands and feet.

Few of us are wholly extrovert or introvert, most of us are a mixture of both types with one or the other predominating; but whether we are mainly gregarious or solitary none of us normally avoids the company of other people altogether. The introvert will not join a boxing club, but he will join a debating society because he wants to exchange ideas with other people. He may dislike the thought of going to a party, but he will spend a lot of time writing letters to friends with the same interests as himself.

Making easy contacts with other people means being flexible in one's approach, wanting to see someone else's point of view, being willing to give one's time and concern to others and realizing that underneath all the differences of money, jobs and background we are all really searching for the same things. Many people hesitate to make the first friendly gesture for fear of being rebuffed or found wanting in some way, only to find that when they finally do so other people respond willingly.

It is a thought worth pondering on that social contacts are made most easily during times of suffering and drama. The supreme example is wartime, when mental illness actually declines and fewer people attempt suicide than during peace, but even a few burst pipes can do more to break down barriers than many a sermon.

To be able to make satisfactory social contacts with other people adds much to the richness and interest of life and gives us a feeling of mutual support, of sharing and of being needed.

LEISURE

Closely connected with our ability to mix easily with others is our enjoyment of leisure. It has been said that the happy man is the man whose work is his hobby, who actually gets paid for doing what he would in any case choose to do in his spare time; but for most of us our work, however enjoyable, is not broad enough to exercise all our abilities. There are facets of our personality which have not found expression in the office or the shop and it is during our leisure that we put this right.

Much daily work is repetitive or routine in nature and a pastime which gives variety and scope for creative ability will bring us increased satisfaction. People who work indoors all day enjoy outdoor sports at the weekend, while the milkman out in all weathers and by himself for most of the day, may enjoy going to a club in the evening and just talking to other people. Many of us with rather dull jobs enjoy the self-expression to be found in amateur theatricals.

For many people adjustment to the demands of sex will always be difficult and pleasure from work, friends and leisure therefore becomes all the more imporant.

With increasing automation and shorter hours, work for most of us may well come to take up a much smaller part of our day and may perhaps become increasingly routine. We shall have more and more spare time, time in which to become depressed and moody, without purpose or satisfaction, or time in which to develop hitherto unknown talents, to meet other people in a meaningful relationship and to discover some of those aspects of life which up to now have been closed to us.

Many mentally ill people have lost the ability to make friends or to find pleasure in work and play. One of the important skills a nurse can learn is the art of helping them to find this pleasure again.

2

Causes and common features of mental illness

We are all born with a certain constitution which belongs to us individually and helps to make us the sort of people we are. This is passed on to us by our parents, through heredity. It may include characteristics from our grandparents and all the ancestors who have gone before us.

A person's constitution is made up of his personality—quick tempered or placid, a thinker or a doer; his physical characteristics—short or tall, rounded or angular; and his intelligence.

From the moment we are born we are subject to influences from our surroundings, the sort of place in which we live, the care or lack of care we receive as children, the attitude of our parents towards us, the neighbourhood in which we are brought up, our teachers and schoolfellows. All these things together form our environment.

As an individual grows from babyhood through childhood to adolescence, he meets many situations of conflict. He has to face his feelings of love and hate towards his mother, he has to learn to behave as society expects even when this stops him from doing something that gives him pleasure. He has to share his mother with his father and with his brothers and sisters although he fears

16

that this sharing will mean less love for him. He has to face the first step away from the security of home which going to school means and then accept the discipline and competition of school life. Until in adolescence he has to become strong enough to step free of his parents and live as a person in his own right, without either the dependence or the rebellion of childhood.

In all these situations he finds himself in a conflict of emotions.

He wants his parents' love and approval but at the same time he feels an urge to do things which he knows will displease them. He wants to follow his own way and yet fears to lose the security of home.

As a child he will try out different ways of getting over these conflicts. He may storm and rage and if this gets him what he wants he will try the same tactics next time. Sometimes blaming someone else works quite well: 'It wasn't me, it was Jimmy Brown'—'You're always getting at me'—'I don't have a chance!' He may find that he can play mother off against father, enlisting sympathy first from one and then from another. Being ill is another way—'Mummy, I don't feel well' often brings everyone running. Perhaps a threat seems the best way—'I'll run away', he says, 'and then you'll all be sorry.' Or he may decide that the best thing is to forget all about what he wants himself and do only what his parents and teachers want. This way he must surely win their approval.

We have all behaved like this many times and it is perfectly normal for children to do so. In the give and take of ordinary family life a child learns to take the rough with the smooth, to come to terms with other people and to grow into a normal, healthy adult who enjoys life.

But adult life does not see the end of conflict. It is not usually the great disasters in life that cause us the most unhappiness. These are more likely to bring us all together. It is the problems that are there as we wake up each morning, when we feel we are left alone to cope by ourselves; problems that other people seem to take in their stride so that we feel we must be rather inferior in some way because we find them difficult. These are the times when we experience stress and as we look around us we can see what some of them are.

MARRIAGE

Two young people are getting married. They want very much to be together and most of the time they are sure it will work out all right, but sometimes they wonder, 'Am I making a mistake?' He listens to his bachelor friends and thinks of the freedom he is giving up, the money it will take to run a home. She wonders whether she will be able to cope with the housework and a job. What will it be like to have a baby? Is he really the right man for her?

Wedding nerves are very common and most couples get over them, but sometimes one or the other falls ill, or backs out with excuses, or runs back to mother.

HAVING CHILDREN

She is going to have a baby. After the first delight at the news the couple settles down to the long time of waiting. Minor inconveniences arise, but they are carried along by the thought that everything will be wonderful when the baby arrives. And so it is for a while.

Then she begins to find nappies and feeding and disturbed nights a wearing business, and to make it worse her husband seems not to notice how much extra work she has to do. She has left her job and misses the companionship of friends at work. She feels tired, bored and sick of being tied to the house.

He, on the other hand, although he is immensely proud of his son and thinks he's a fine little chap, begins

18

to feel rather left out in the cold. It's all baby, baby, baby! She seems to have no time for him nowadays. When he comes home she's too tired to talk about anything—except, of course, the baby—and she doesn't bother to look as pretty as she used to do. They had so looked forward to this and now the baby is spoiling it all.

Without realizing it he is beginning to feel as jealous as he did when he was three years old and his baby brother arrived on the scene at home.

Fortunately nappies come to an end at last, a sense of humour and proportion comes to their aid and most parents can share their feelings with each other, drawing closer than they were before as a result. But for a few their life together may never be quite as good again. For some women the physical and psychological effect of childbirth itself will bring on a mental illness.

CHILDREN LEAVING HOME

The children grow up and go out to work. Then they, too, get married and leave home. 'We'll do that later on, when the children are off our hands.' How often had the parents said this in the past, when life was so full. Now the children really have gone and life stretches out ahead, long and empty. They have all the time in the world but somehow it seems a little flat and nothing is worth doing now that they have at last come to it.

It takes an effort to make a new life again, to find as much interest and purpose as they had when their time was so occupied by the children, and some find it easier to slip down into apathy and depression.

CHANGE OF LIFE

The menopause, the time when a woman stops having her periods, is a time of considerable adjustment for her, both physically and emotionally. She may feel unusually tired, have headaches and dizzy spells, or she may have no symptoms at all, but inevitably she realizes that she is losing one of her main functions as a woman, that of being able to bear children. Unconsciously she may feel that because she is no longer able to have a baby she will be less attractive to her husband.

Most women pass through this stage without difficulty. They are already leading a full and happy life and they continue to do so, secure in the love of family and friends, but to others it can be a time of severe stress and it is not uncommon for women to become mentally ill at this time. Fortunately this kind of mental illness can easily be cured.

Many people do not realize that men may also go through a similar time of difficulty when they begin to realize that their sexual powers are decreasing.

RETIREMENT

Retirement from the work they have done all their lives brings many problems to both men and women.

There may be money worries. Perhaps the pension is small and it means moving into a flat or a room where the rent is less and cutting down on luxuries and extras. Making friends is not so easy in a new district and old contacts are lost. Holidays are less frequent. The days which were once so busy are not only empty, but lonely too. Work had its drawbacks but there was always someone to share them with. He remembers the jokes in the canteen. She misses the gossip and backchat when there were a few minutes to spare. But above all there is the thought, quickly pushed away, that one is no longer of any use, getting too old for it, thrown on the scrap heap.

Again this is a time of stress calling for considerable adjustment. Many people literally start a new life after retirement, developing skills which amaze and delight their friends, but others less well balanced may need help.

OLD AGE

Finally in old age we face again some of the problems of infancy, the fear of being helpless, the frustration of being dependent on others for the satisfaction of our needs. The longing for warmth and affection. There is also the loss of loved ones through death, the fear of death for ourselves and the despair that comes from knowing one is no longer of use to anyone else, or even worse of knowing that one is a burden to those one loves. In the right circumstances old age can be tranquil, serene and sunny, but too often it is clouded with depression and regrets.

It is very true that babies need loving into this world and old people need loving out.

These and many other difficulties come to all of us and we tend to fall back on the old ways of behaving that we tried as a child, particularly those that we found worked well. We run away, or we develop all sorts of aches and pains, or we say it is not our fault, and someone else is getting at us, or we burst into tears. We clothe them in adult words and actions of course, but the pattern is the same.

This is perfectly normal provided we don't do it all the time. We may all react inappropriately on occasions, but if we go on doing so it becomes abnormal.

For instance, a man's wife tells him the dog from next door has broken the fence down and what is he going to do about it she wants to know. He may say that he has had a tiring day at the office and doesn't feel well enough to do anything about it, or he may decide to tell his other neighbours, hoping they will take the matter up on his behalf. He may go and have a stand-up row with the dog's owner; on the other hand he may refuse to speak to him next time he sees him. Or, of course, he may settle the matter in a friendly chat over a pint of beer.

Each of these actions is normal, but if after a year has gone by he is still not speaking to his neighbour, or if he is still telling other people all about it, then this is an abnormal reaction to stress.

When our abnormal reaction to stress becomes so pronounced that it prevents us from leading our everyday lives, we are said to be suffering from mental illness.

The causes of mental illness are not yet fully understood, but the following factors are thought to be involved.

ORGANIC DISEASE

Physical illness which affects the brain, such as hardening of the arteries (arteriosclerosis), or a high fever, may cause mental symptoms. For example, an elderly man with arteriosclerosis may lose his memory and become confused. He may wander about the house at night and not recognize his wife and children. Someone in a high fever may become delirious or see things around him which, in fact, are not there.

HEREDITY

Some psychiatrists think mental illness may be inherited. Certain mental illnesses run in families, but much more research is needed before we can say definitely whether this is so or not.

CONSTITUTION AND ENVIRONMENT

Our constitution, our relationships with our parents and our childhood experiences play a big part because our emotional struggles in infancy have set a pattern for our reaction to later difficulties and we tend to go on reacting in this way when we are adults. If our pattern in childhood was unsatisfactory we shall be more likely to react in an abnormal way when we grow up.

PSYCHOLOGICAL STRESS

Difficulties in connection with work, sexual relationships, family affairs or social life may precipitate mental illness, but what is a catastrophe or an intolerable burden to one person may simply spur another on to greater efforts. It depends on where our weakness lies.

A man lost his business and all his savings in a financial crash. He started with nothing and built it all up again, only to become ill when his wife left him for another man.

A woman who nursed her invalid mother for many years with great devotion became ill when her mother finally died and left her alone.

Each one of us, however well balanced, will break down if the pressure is great enough. We can think of mental illness as a persistently abnormal way of reacting to the difficulties which we all experience, or as a means of getting away from a situation which has become too much for us to bear.

The more we understand and accept our own feelings the stronger we shall be and the more we shall be able to help others.

Mental illnesses can be divided into two large groups, the neuroses and the psychoses.

A neurotic is suffering from a disorder of his emotions. A psychotic is suffering from a disorder of the mind itself.

We all behave in a neurotic way at times. This is quite normal. It is when our neurotic behaviour persists that we need the help of a doctor. For example:

Normal   However does Mrs. Jones keep her curtains so white! I really must wash mine next week.

Neurotic   I clean the house from top to bottom every day

and still it looks dirty. I'm too exhausted to do any more.

Psychotic   I am unclean. I have poisoned the whole world and God is destroying me as a punishment.

The neurotic believes something which is possible, but not probable. The psychotic believes something which is quite impossible.

Normal   So Roberts got the job? Oh well, I suppose my face just didn't fit.

Neurotic   It's always the same. Jealous! That's what they are. I should have been promoted long ago, but they're just determined to see I don't get on. They gang up against me each time.

Psychotic   The Government knows I have the secret formula which will split the earth in two. Their agents are following me everywhere. You're one of them—you can't fool me.

The neurotic can be brought to see that he is ill, although he does not always agree with the doctor about the cause of his illness. The psychotic cannot see that he is ill. There are exceptions to this rule, but it is true in most instances.

Normal   Don't tell me the lift is out of order again! Oh well, I'd rather walk up the stairs than get stuck in the lift. That must be very unpleasant.

Neurotic   I can't bear to be shut in anywhere. I can't even stay in a room if the door is shut. It's silly, I know. Yes, I suppose it is a kind of illness. I only wish I could get over it.

Psychotic   I'm the strongest man in the world. I could knock the roof off this place with one hand if I wanted to. You can't keep me in anywhere! No, of course I'm not ill. It's you miserable devils who are only half alive. Don't come bothering me now, I'm counting the stars.

The main neuroses are Anxiety neurosis
Obsessive-compulsive neurosis
Hysteria

The psychoses can be further divided into those in which physical disease plays a major part and those in which it does not. These subdivisions are called organic psychoses and functional psychoses.

The main organic
psychoses are   Dementia
Infective-exhaustive
psychoses

The functional psychoses
are   Schizophrenia
Manic-depressive psychoses

ANXIETY NEUROSIS

We all know what it is to feel anxious. Anxiety becomes abnormal when it is out of all proportion to the cause, or when it continues long after the cause has been removed.

Patients with other mental illnesses often feel anxious from time to time, but the term anxiety neurosis is used to describe the illness in which anxiety is the main feature and the patient feels anxious all the time.

OBSESSIVE-COMPULSIVE NEUROSIS

Some people will not walk under a ladder, a few would be really worried if you forced them to do so. They are obsessed by the thought that it is unlucky. Some people feel compelled to throw spilt salt over their shoulders.

If a person is obsessed by a thought to such an extent, or compelled to perform certain actions so frequently that he is unable to lead a normal life he is suffering from obsessive-compulsive neurosis. The obsessions and compulsions take many different forms. The patient knows they are unreasonable but he is unable to control them. One of the most common compulsions is the need to wash time and time again, another is extreme tidiness.

HYSTERIA

The popular meaning of the word 'hysterical' is out of control, as in 'she became hysterical', meaning she started screaming uncontrollably or laughing and crying at the same time.

In medical language the word is used to mean that a symptom is beyond the patient's control.

If I have to take an examination tomorrow and to get out of it I ring up to say I cannot attend because I am going to the dentist, I am malingering. I am quite deliberately telling a lie to get out of taking the examination. But if, on the morning of the examination, I wake up with a raging toothache although there is nothing wrong with my tooth, this is hysteria. There is nothing wrong, but the pain is excrutiatingly genuine. I am quite truly incapable of sitting an examination. The symptom is out of my conscious control and has become hysterical.

Hysterical symptoms always serve to get us out of some unpleasant situation, to gain us some advantage, or to solve some conflict for us. People in whom hysterical symptoms are so pronounced that they can no longer lead an ordinary life are said to be suffering from hysteria.

DEMENTIA

This is the mental illness associated with decay or deterioration of the brain. It usually occurs in people over sixty, but occasionally earlier. In old people it is called senile dementia.

Most old people retain their faculties quite well, but sometimes the brain ages and becomes diseased while the body remains comparatively healthy. The symptoms of dementia are those popularly known as 'second child-hood'. The patient forgets the immediate past but re-members his early life clearly. He doesn't recognize people he knows well, frequently forgets where he has put things, doesn't know where he is or what day it is. Small changes in his routine make him confused. He is unable to grasp any new ideas. Sometimes he is ex-tremely obstinate and at others quite docile.

INFECTIVE-EXHAUSTIVE PSYCHOSIS

Physical illnesses which are accompanied by infection or exhaustion sometimes give rise to mental symptoms.

The most common is puerperal septicaemia or infec-tion following childbirth. Others are pneumonia, in-fluenza, tuberculosis, cancer and some diseases of the nervous system. The patient is restless, sleeps little and when he does he has vivid dreams which he believes are real. He cannot think clearly and does not know what is going on. He sees and hears what is not there, may lose his memory and is often incoherent and noisy. He lives half in this world and half in a dream world.

SCHIZOPHRENIA

This is the most common of the psychoses and the most difficult to understand. There are different types of schizophrenia and symptoms may vary from being moody and difficult to the most bizarre thoughts and actions.

The patient may hear voices and see things which are not there. This is called being hallucinated. He thinks in a way that is incomprehensible to normal people. He may hold beliefs which to ordinary people around him are quite untenable, such as that his arms are stuffed with cotton wool. Such beliefs are called delusions. He often thinks that everything which happens refers to him and that other people are conspiring against him. He is sometimes excited and at others apathetic or stuporose and is given to acting suddenly, without warning.

The popular term 'split mind', although not accurate, may have come from the way in which these patients will laugh as they describe some dreadful happening which they believe has just taken place, as if their emotions had been split off and no longer worked in harmony with their thoughts.

MANIC-DEPRESSIVE PSYCHOSIS

We all know what it is like to feel depressed. Depression is perhaps the easiest mental illness to understand, because it is so clearly an exaggeration of what everyone goes through at times.

Depression which is so deep that it prevents a person from living an ordinary life, or makes him think of committing suicide, is a mental illness.

Sometimes we can recognize the cause of our depression. Perhaps someone we love has died, or our employer has given us notice. Feelings of depression in these circumstances are natural. If they develop into a mental illness it will be known as a reactive depression, because we are reacting against something which happened to us, in this case the death of a loved one or the loss of our job.

Sometimes depression settles like a cloud for no obvious reason at all. If this kind of depression develops into a mental illness it is called an endogenous depression, meaning one which comes from within the person himself, not from outside.

Women sometimes suffer from a depressive illness at the time of the menopause and this is known as involutional depression. A similar depression may affect men between the ages of fifty and sixty.

The opposite to depression is feeling on top of the world,

and happily we all know what this is like too, when all we have planned goes well and we are on good terms with the world.

We know too that there are times when we fill our lives with ceaseless activity, running from one task to another, always animated and full of bright ideas, ready to try anything for a new diversion. The radio is on all day. We must have someone with us, and we chatter non-stop. We can't stand silence, or having nothing to do, and we don't go to bed until we are too tired to lie awake and think.

This is not feeling on top of the world. It is more like whistling in the dark. When we do stop for a moment we know that all our activity is really an effort to avoid thinking about how depressed we feel. This also is natural, but if the constant activity becomes so pronounced that we are incapable of carrying on an ordinary life we are said to be suffering from mania.

Among the patients in a psychiatric hospital you will find a few who are suffering from mania, a great many whose illness is depression, and one or two in whom mania and depression alternate in a regular pattern.

3

How patients get treatment

The National Health Service for England and Wales, which came into operation in 1948, provides medical and social services for all kinds of illness. The Mental Health Services are that part of the National Health Service which helps people who are mentally disordered.

One in four adults suffer from psychiatric symptoms. One woman in every nine and one man in every fourteen will spend some time in a psychiatric hospital during their lifetimes. One hundred people kill themselves every week in Britain and 400 more try to do so.

There was a time when to have tuberculosis was considered a shameful thing. It was something you tried to hide from the neighbours. People with tuberculosis thought they were being punished for some sin. Parents and relatives felt as guilty as if they had committed a crime. It was said to be a judgement on the family.

Today no one would think for a moment that a patient suffering from tuberculosis was wicked or that his family had done something dreadful.

Children and young people rarely develop tuberculosis now, mainly because we understand the importance of keeping them really healthy. If they do show signs of having the disease it is noticed quickly and treatment is prompt and thorough.

More and more people today are coming to see that

this attitude holds good for mental health as well as physical health and the old prejudice against mental illness is beginning to disappear.

THE GENERAL PRACTITIONER

When Mr G feels physically ill he goes to see his doctor at his surgery or telephones and asks his doctor to come and see him. If he cannot do this for himself a relative or friend will do it for him.

The same thing happens if he becomes mentally ill. His general practitioner will see him during surgery hours, or if he is too ill to come to the surgery will visit him at home.

OUTPATIENT TREATMENT

If the illness is mild and the general practitioner has been told about it at an early stage it is quite possible that he will treat it himself, just as he would if Mr G had an attack of influenza. The fact that he has been called in at the first sign of illness is important because it prevents complications and hastens the rate of recovery in mental illness just as it does with physical complaints.

On the other hand Mr G's doctor may decide that he would like him to be seen by a specialist. In this case he will make an appointment for him to attend the outpatients' department at the district hospital. Here he will be seen in the psychiatric clinic by a consultant psychiatrist—a doctor who specializes in mental illness.

The psychiatrist may say that he would like Mr G to come up and see him in the outpatients' department once or twice a week for a while, just as the consultant physician might want to see him if he had diabetes or the orthopaedic surgeon might ask him to attend the fracture clinic if he had broken his leg.

This may be all that is needed and Mr G will continue to go to work in the ordinary way, his employers giving him time off to attend the clinic when necessary, until he has recovered.

HOSPITAL TREATMENT

However, the psychiatrist may feel that it would be better for Mr G to come into hospital. In this case he will arrange for him to be admitted to the psychiatric unit of the district hospital, or to a psychiatric hospital.

A psychiatric unit is a group of wards in a district hospital. The psychiatric unit specializes in one type of illness, namely mental illness. There are, of course, other special units in general hospitals, such as the intensive care unit or the neurosurgical unit.

Whichever hospital Mr G goes into his stay is not likely to be a long one. Seventy per cent of the people admitted for mental illness are sent home in less than three months and many within six weeks.

While in hospital Mr G will be able to have as many visits from friends and relatives as he likes and he is likely also to spend several weekends at home before he is finally discharged.

If Mr G is too ill to go to the outpatients' department his general practitioner may ask the consultant psychiatrist to come and see him in his own home, as he might for example ask a heart specialist to visit a patient at home. The consultant will then come and examine him and offer his advice in the usual way.

Of course Mr G may refuse to take the advice his doctors give him. In this case nothing can be done unless Mr G's illness is of such a nature that his doctor is concerned for his safety or for the safety of other people. For example, Mr G may say that he intends to kill himself as soon as he can, or his doctor may have reason to believe that Mr G is planning to harm his neighbours. If this is so he may arrange for Mr G to be taken to hospital in spite of the fact that he does not wish to go.

A drowning man will often struggle so hard with his rescuer that he has to be brought ashore against his will as it were, and something of the same principle is at work with compulsory admissions to hospital. Very few people need to be admitted in this way. The procedures connected with compulsory admission are discussed in Chapter Twenty-one on 'Legal Matters'.

CARE OF PATIENT'S HOME

If Mr G was living alone before he went into hospital and has no friend or relative who can look after his affairs the social worker in the hospital, with Mr G's permission, will get in touch with the area health authority in his district. They will see that one of their own social workers looks after Mr G's home and gets everything ready for him when he is discharged.

NIGHT HOSTELS

When the time comes for Mr G to leave hospital he may go straight home if he has a wife and family waiting to welcome him.

If, however, he is alone his doctor may think it best for him to go at first to a night hostel, run by the area health authority. These are houses offering accommodation for a small group of patients who can treat it as their home and yet be in touch with nursing and medical help if necessary.

The patients go out to work during the day and return in the evening to the hostel, where they spend the night. A member of the staff is always on duty and a doctor can be called if necessary. In this way the patients can get accustomed to work and everyday life gradually, knowing that there is someone in the background ready to listen and support them if they feel doubtful.

After a few weeks in the hostel Mr G will feel ready to

look after himself again and will return to his own room or flat, which the social worker has got ready for him.

RETURNING HOME

Although he is now discharged from hospital help is still freely available to him if he wants it. With his permission the social worker, from the area health authority, will call on him from time to time to see that all is well and to advise him on any problems he may have.

Meanwhile the psychiatrist, who has been looking after Mr G while he was in hospital, will have been in touch with his general practitioner to let him know that Mr G is now home again. When he hears this the general practitioner may go round and see how Mr G is getting on and, if necessary, arrange to supply any medicines Mr G may still be taking.

The psychiatrist will also have made an appointment for Mr G to come and see him at the outpatients' department in a few weeks' time for a check up, just as a surgeon would do if Mr G had been having an operation. In this way skilled help is always at hand until Mr G is back in good health again.

DAY HOSPITALS

Sometimes it is not necessary for patients to be admitted to hospital if there is a day hospital in the district.

The day hospital is run by the main hospital, and patients come during the day for treatment, returning in the evening to their own homes. While at the day hospital they are cared for by nurses and doctors as if they were in a psychiatric unit or psychiatric hospital.

Treatment in a day hospital is particularly suitable for

older people living with relatives who go out to work during the day but are willing to look after the old person at night. Sleeping in their own homes is less confusing for them than being in a strange place. It also helps to maintain the link with relatives and neighbours, which can easily be broken where elderly people are concerned.

Patients may be taken to and from the day hospital each day, either by their relatives or by ambulance. Many are able to make the journey by themselves.

FURTHER ADVICE

These are some of the ways in which people can get treatment under the National Health Service.

Anyone who needs information or advice can go to his general practitioner, who has behind him the full resources of the mental health service and will always be able to help him.

4

The hospital team

Patients come into a psychiatric hospital or a psychiatric unit because they need treatment and can no longer lead a happy and satisfactory life in the outside world.

The aim of the hospital is to help them back to normal life and to a return to the outside world as soon as possible.

For this reason life in a psychiatric hospital or unit is very like life outside, but the hospital is flexible and adjusts itself to the patient's needs in a way that the outside world is not able to do. Here he can feel that he is accepted without criticism, that people want to understand him and that he will get help with his problems.

If patients are to lead as normal a life as possible they will need food, sleep, work, recreation and the company of other people, including those of the opposite sex. The various wards will provide accommodation for eating and sleeping. There will be workshops where patients can learn a trade or develop a hobby, and a large recreation hall which can be used for socials and dances, or adapted as a cinema or theatre.

If their lives while in hospital are, indeed, to be as near normal as possible, it seems reasonable that men and women should carry out these ordinary activities together. To meet this need many hospitals are setting up integrated wards, in which men and women patients are

36

cared for by a mixed staff of men and women nurses. The effect on the patients is often quite marked. Women smarten themselves up, put on a little makeup and take more notice of what is going on around them. Men comb their hair, do up their buttons, swear less and brush up their manners. Both men and women patients seem to find the daily routine a little more interesting when they are sharing in this way. Incidentally, the same observations can often be made about the nurses in a mixed ward.

Doubts as to the desirability of integrated wards are sometimes expressed by patients, their friends and relatives and by nurses too, but in practice these units work well. Of course, no patient should be forced to stay in a mixed ward if he or she dislikes the idea, and some, in any case, would not find such a ward helpful and would be excluded on medical grounds.

Many hospitals have what is known as a social centre or a community centre, where such facilities as a library, a hairdressing salon, rooms for music, games and discussions are conveniently grouped together, often with a well-stocked shop and a café where patients can entertain their visitors.

In a psychiatric hospital or psychiatric unit the work of every single member of the staff has an effect on the patients. Not only the nurses and doctors, but clerks, porters and domestic staff, gardeners, cooks and engineers can all help or hinder the patients' progress. Everything that is done by any member of the staff should be measured against this yardstick—how will it help the patients. So that when we talk of the hospital team we mean everyone on the staff, working in co-operation with one another, towards the same end—the patient's recovery.

The hospital team can be divided into three large groups. These are the nursing staff, the medical staff and the hospital administrative staff.

NURSING STAFF

For administrative purposes most large hospitals are divided into areas, controlled by senior nursing officers. Each area consists of four to six units, a unit being a group of wards under the control of a nursing officer and a senior doctor, known as a consultant. Between them the nursing officer and the consultant plan and organize the nursing and medical services for their unit. Decisions affecting the whole hospital are taken at a higher level and are passed on to the unit nursing officer, who in turn informs the nurses in the wards.

The day-to-day nursing care of the patients is in the hands of the charge nurses. A charge nurse is a qualified nurse in charge of a ward and may be a man or a woman. When the charge nurse is a woman she is often referred to as a ward sister. The number of nurses in a ward will vary according to the patients' needs and the staff available. A busy ward may have a sister or charge nurse, a staff nurse, enrolled nurses, part-time trained nurses and nurses in training. Staff nurses and enrolled nurses are fully trained people whose duty is to assist the sister or charge nurse and to deputize for him in his absence. Nurses in training may be people who have never done nursing before, or they may be general trained nurses who are learning psychiatric nursing.

The training of nurses is organized by the teaching division of the hospital and the nurses working here are called tutors. A tutor is a senior nurse who has had a university training to qualify him, or her, as a teacher of nursing. Tutors devote the whole of their time to the education of nurses in training and are especially concerned with the theoretical aspect of the training. They also organize in-service courses for trained nurses and are consulted on, or assist in, other educational activities in the hospital. In the wards they are helped by the nursing

38

officers, the charge nurses and also by the clinical teachers who are trained nurses with an extra qualification in the art of ward teaching.

There are always some members of the nursing staff on duty night and day and because of their close contact with the patients, they play a vital part in their treatment. In every hospital the trained nursing staff are some of the most important members of the hospital team. This is why the senior nursing officers are so often asked for advice on matters connected with nursing and much of their time may be spent preparing reports, attending committees and discussing problems or new ideas with other departments.

The nursing officers, senior nursing officers and tutors are together known as the administrative nursing staff.

MEDICAL STAFF

The senior doctors are the consultants and one of them will be appointed as the medical administrator for the hospital. He may be known as the medical director, or as the chairman of the medical committee, but in each case he acts as spokesman for his fellow doctors on all occasions when their advice is needed.

As with the nursing administrator, his help is constantly needed, not only over such obvious items as medical equipment or drugs, but with all the manifold decisions that have to be made in the administration of a large community.

Everything that happens in a psychiatric hospital affects the patients to a greater or lesser degree, whether it be altering the nurses' hours of duty, building a new ward, or changing the laundry arrangements. Because of this there is close co-operation between doctors, nurses and hospital administrative staff, and changes are fully discussed on all sides before the go-ahead is given.

The doctor's work is to diagnose the patient's illness

39

and decide on the best treatment for him. Part of the treatment he will carry out himself and part will be in the hands of nurses and other specialist staff.

The consultants and junior doctors are assisted in their work by a number of specially trained people, among them the social worker, the psychologist and the occupational therapist.

The social worker is concerned with the patient's family background, his job and his social problems. When Mary R came into the hospital in a very depressed state the social worker was able to tell the doctor that Mary and her husband John had four children, all under seven, that they were living in two rooms and that John drank heavily. This helped the doctor a great deal when he was talking to Mary about her difficulties. While Mary was in hospital the social worker arranged for John to have help with the children and when his wife was discharged from hospital she helped them both to start afresh.

The psychologist is trained to understand people's behaviour and to detect when it is abnormal. He can test patients in ways that will help the doctor to find out what is wrong. When Mary was admitted she seemed to be rather stupid and it was difficult to tell whether it was her depression which made her seem like this or whether she was really below average in intelligence. The psychologist tested her mental ability and was able to tell the doctor that it was in fact slightly above the average. The psychologist can also advise on the choice of a career, or on a change of work, and he plays an important part in research into such matters as ways of selecting staff, or the relative value of various methods of treatment.

We all need to express ourselves in some way, to make something, whether it be a symphony, a new dress, or a happy family, and the occupational therapist helps patients gain confidence by discovering new ways of using their abilities. Mary had difficulty in making both ends meet on the money left over after John's drinking bouts. In the occupational therapy department she joined a homecraft group where she found a new interest, and a way of saving money by learning to make some of her own clothes. Occupational therapists also help with the organizing of social and recreational activities in the hospital.

Another person whose work is closely connected with that of both doctors and nurses is the pharmacist. He is responsible for the ordering, safe-keeping and dispensing of all drugs and medical preparations used in the hospital. The pharmacist can give much helpful information to the doctors and nurses about the use of drugs, which in many cases is controlled by law.

HOSPITAL ADMINISTRATIVE STAFF

Since the National Health Service reorganization most psychiatric hospitals have become part of a district, consisting of a variety of different types of hospitals. The district is administered by a district management team and the individual hospitals have administrative staff who all report to the district management team.

Running a hospital is a costly business, and the bills are the responsibility of the district finance officer. Just as a family will budget for food, heat, light, repairs, clothes and entertainment, so he budgets for the hospital. A family will get together and talk over how to spend its money and in the same way he discusses the hospital budget with the heads of the various departments in the hospital. He keeps all the accounts and pays all the bills. Quite the largest bill he has to pay each year consists of wages and salaries for all the staff in the hospital, including of course the nursing staff.

The head of the supplies department is responsible for seeing that everything the other departments need is available at the time they need it and in the quantities needed. He makes sure that the money is spent as economically as possible and that the hospital gets good value. His store may hold as great a variety as any market square—ballpoint pens, bales of curtain material, sacks of potatoes, crates of cups and saucers, table cloths and tennis balls, detergents and sealing wax—all kept together like treasure in Aladdin's Cave.

The heating, lighting and plumbing of the hospital are the responsibility of the engineers. They are as proud of their great boilers and as knowledgeable about them as any motor racing enthusiast about the latest models on the track. It is the engineers who give the hospital all the pleasure that comes from bright lights on a dark night, ice cubes in a heatwave and constant hot water all the year round.

A psychiatric hospital may have accommodation for anything between 500 and 2000 patients, or more, and this means a large number of buildings of different kinds. The task of keeping all these walls and ceilings in repair, painting and decorating, mending that broken sash cord and replacing the tiles that came down in last night's gale is the responsibility of the building staff. Some of the buildings may be nearly 100 years old and the engineers and building staff between them are performing miracles of modernization, so that what were once huge dark wards are now bright, attractive and friendly.

A very important subject from everyone's point of view is the food service for the hospital. A nice cup of tea in front of the fire, turkey at Christmas and hot cross buns at Easter, strawberries for Sports Day and roast beef on Sundays, all this is the work of the chef and kitchen staff, not to mention good, wholesome food four times a day for perhaps 2500 people.

The cleanliness of the hospital is taken care of by the domestic staff. It is their responsibility to supply domestic help for every ward and department in the hospital. Not an easy task when there is a shortage of staff and buildings are old, but vitally important, especially in the wards

The hospital team

where help with the domestic work can free the nursing staff to spend more time with the patients.

The function of the hospital administrative staff is to provide the setting in which patients can receive the specialized help of the doctors and nurses. In addition to those mentioned above there are many others who contribute in this way. The staff in the records office, who look after reports on discharged patients, the porters and laundry staff, the typists and telephonists, all are essential to the smooth running of the community which is the hospital.

Together these three groups of staff, nursing, medical and hospital administrative, form the hospital team, and as in any team if the members work together, understanding each other's contribution to the whole, the power of the team is far greater than when each one works on his own regardless of the others.

The nursing officers know every department in the hospital and may be in the occupational therapy room or the engineers' workshop as often as they are in the wards, while the charge nurse may find himself consulting the catering department or the domestic staff almost as often as he does the ward doctors.

In the ward itself charge nurse and the other nurses will talk over the patient's progress and plan further treatment with the doctor, the social worker and the occupational therapist, often with the help of the tutors and administrative nursing staff who visit the wards regularly.

In this way it is possible for the hospital team to develop its full potential and bring real healing to the patients in its care.

5

Rehabilitation

When a patient comes into hospital he hands his problems over to the hospital team and waits to be cured, not thinking that any further effort is required of him.

The work of the team is to cure or relieve his illness and to build up his personality so that he can either deal with his problems himself, or lead a life as satisfying as possible in spite of them.

This is called rehabilitation. It used to be thought that rehabilitation applied only to patients who had been in hospital a long time. It is now coming to be widely accepted that not only these patients, but every patient, from the moment he is admitted to hospital, needs rehabilitation in one form or another. Individual treatment will vary according to the particular illness, but all patients need rehabilitating to a greater or lesser degree.

Rehabilitation may be achieved in two ways:

1. Through a therapeutic community which encourages the patient to take an active part in his recovery.
2. Through a programme of planned activity which restores his independence and his ability to accept responsibility for his own actions.

THERAPEUTIC COMMUNITY

A therapeutic community is, literally, a community which promotes healing.

The hospital team cannot 'make' patients better. Mental health cannot be imposed on them like a traffic regulation, or offered to them like a dose of medicine. But it may begin to grow if patients can form good relationships with other people. This means that if the hospital is to be a therapeutic community staff and patients must together form relationships which will help the patient's recovery. Two conditions are necessary if this is to happen.

Firstly, communications throughout the hospital should be as open as possible. Everyone must feel that he can say what he thinks and that he is free to offer suggestions to others. This applies to patients with each other, to patients with staff, and to members of the staff with each other.

Secondly, antisocial behaviour should be accepted and an attempt made to understand its meaning.

In the past, when patients behaved in a way not acceptable in ordinary society, the first thought in the minds of the staff was 'He mustn't do that—what can we do to stop him?' Today the thought is 'What is he trying to tell us by his behaviour?'

Each hospital develops its own way of establishing a therapeutic community. Details vary from one to another, but the following methods are practised in many hospitals.

WARD OR UNIT MEETINGS

These are meetings of all the patients and all the staff connected with the ward or unit. A typical meeting might include patients, nurses, the ward or unit doctor, occupational therapists, a social worker, perhaps a nursing officer and a tutor, and sometimes the ward maid.

The size of the group will, of course, depend on the number of patients in the ward or unit and will vary a good deal. Most ward meetings are held in the morning, but they can just as well take place later if this suits members better. Discussion usually goes on for about an hour. Chairs are placed in a large circle because this is more informal than sitting in rows one behind another. There are no special seats for staff. They mix with the patients and sit wherever there happens to be an empty chair.

The first ward meetings are usually in the nature of grumble sessions—'Can we have more sugar at tea time?', 'Some people leave the baths dirty', 'Do we have to go to bed before television ends?', and so on. Many practical problems come up and if the staff are willing to listen to the patients and see their point of view improvements may be worked out which make life more pleasant for everyone.

Some hospitals go no further than this. They hold ward meetings once a week or once a fortnight and use them to sort out the domestic and administrative problems in the ward. This is helpful, but it fails to develop the full possibilities of the situation. The everyday problems are gradually solved and there is nothing more to talk about. Staff get bored and think it is a waste of time. This attitude is picked up by the patients and meetings are only called when there is some specific complaint to discuss.

Other hospitals find that if they persevere with frequent meetings patients can be encouraged to talk not only about day to day complaints but about their own feelings as well.

The extent to which they can do this will depend almost entirely on the staff's attitude. Many of the problems which occur may involve criticism of the ward or unit team. The patients who ask for more sugar may really be thinking 'Why is there always plenty when Charge Nurse A is on duty, but Charge Nurse B never lets us have enough?' The comment about going to bed before the television programme has finished might mean 'We think Nurse C is too bossy.'

If they put their feelings into words in this way it is natural for the staff concerned to become anxious and to start justifying their actions. 'I can't give you what isn't there, can I?' or 'You know the rule is bed at ten o'clock'.

Faced with this kind of response patients may soon stop talking, but if the staff can refrain from immediately justifying themselves discussion may develop along more helpful lines.

Perhaps there is a certain amount of rivalry between Charge Nurse A's shift and Charge Nurse B's which leads, among other things, to discrepancies in the allocation of supplies. On the other hand it may be that the patient who made the remark would like to see a rift developing between Charge Nurse A and Charge Nurse B. Why should this give him satisfaction? What relationship is he trying to establish between himself and the two nurses?

Perhaps Nurse C *is* too bossy. Or maybe she is scared of Miss D the night sister, who always expects patients to be in bed when she comes into the ward. Perhaps the patient who wanted to stay up beyond his bedtime would like to defy Nurse C's authority and is trying to get the others to side with him against her. On the other hand perhaps it would be helpful to review the evening routine and consider whether patients could go to bed later on special occasions.

If this kind of discussion is possible the ward or unit meeting becomes a setting in which patients can try out relationships with the staff and with each other. They have a need to talk over their difficulties together and if the staff do not intervene too much they will often answer each other. In this way they can begin to understand some of the reasons behind their faulty relationships and learn to change them.

Patients respond much more to acceptance and understanding than to rigid discipline, which may only reinforce their antisocial attitudes.

Staff who feel able to allow real freedom of speech usually find that they achieve the best results by holding meetings three or four times a week. In this way impetus is maintained and a sense of real community develops among patients and staff.

Generally no particular subject is chosen for discussion. Everyone is free to say what comes into his mind. If a particular incident has caused anxiety or the staff have an administrative problem which is worrying them they may bring it up, and similarly patients can talk about anything that is causing them concern.

All changes will be discussed at these meetings before being carried out. This is helpful first of all from a practical point of view because others in the group may be able to draw attention to factors which had not been taken into account, or suggest modifications which will improve the scheme. It also increases the feeling of mutual trust and confidence between staff and patients. If changes are made without this sharing the patients feel badly let down and will say 'Why weren't we told? What's wrong? Don't they trust us?' The therapeutic relationship is broken. Patients withdraw into themselves again and their symptoms increase.

Attendance at meetings is not compulsory but the doctor makes it clear to patients that the unit meeting is part of their treatment and that he expects them to be there. The attitude of the nurses also has an effect. If they think the meetings are important the patients will think so too and attendance will be high.

In some wards many of the patients may be too apathetic, too withdrawn or preoccupied to say what they are feeling. They may remain quite silent. But if meetings are held frequently they come to realize that the staff are trying to understand their difficulties and in turn are trying to share their own problems with the patients. This builds up a climate of appreciation and trust and the process of drawing the patient back from his world of fantasy becomes a little less difficult.

STAFF MEETINGS

Following each meeting the ward or unit team meets together for half an hour, usually over a cup of coffee, to talk over what has been happening in the ward meeting. Again the meeting is quite informal and everyone is free to speak.

For many members of the staff the ward meeting can be a disturbing experience. It is not easy to be criticized by the patients if you are the junior nurse and your charge nurse or the nursing officer is present. Nor does charge nurse or sister always appreciate having her authority questioned in front of the occupational therapist or the ward doctor. Patients can be irritating and you may find it hard to keep your temper. Perhaps you have always done your best to carry out charge nurse's instructions and then someone in the meeting makes you feel thoroughly silly, so that you begin to wonder what really is the right thing to do.

The staff meeting is held so that members may share the anxieties and problems raised by the ward meeting and help each other to understand what has been going on. It is a relief to discover that you are not the only one who finds Mr D so annoying, or that some of the others are also disgusted by Mrs E's behaviour. The occupational therapist may be glad of the chance to talk about something that made her feel angry in the ward meeting, and the doctor may want everyone's opinion on a new line of treatment he thinks may be helpful. You will be able to tell charge nurse that you are confused about what you should be doing and in the discussion that follows some of the problems will be straightened out.

The ward meeting and the staff meeting together form the nucleus of the therapeutic community. Each is dependent on the other and neither is completely effective without the other. The names given to the meetings will vary from hospital to hospital, but the aim, to promote therapeutic relationships through free discussion, remains the same.

Usually the ward or unit doctor leads both meetings, but occasionally he may not be able to attend and the charge nurse or nursing officer will take his place.

PATIENTS' GROUPS

Through discussion in the ward meetings the patient begins to see that he has not come into hospital to sit back passively and wait to be cured. Getting better is an active process in which he has to play his part just as much as the staff have to play theirs.

To carry this process a stage further patients meet in small groups by themselves. They undertake such tasks as organizing social activities or planning the day's work in the ward.

In order to do these things successfully they have to make a start at dealing with their own problems and helping others in the group to do the same. For instance, some people always like to be in the limelight, but in any project there must always be many who have to do humdrum jobs compared with the one or two who get the applause. Those who want the praise must come to terms with each other and with the rest of the group about who is going to do what.

Other patients may feel shy and unable to contribute anything. For them the group may be a support. A small job can usually be found which they will be able to tackle. Later on, when they know the others better, they may be able to talk about how they feel.

Some of us do not like being told what to do, but have

no objection to telling others. This is not always welcomed. The group provides an opportunity for patients to try out different kinds of leadership and to discuss why some of them may feel angry with each other. The ward team is always at hand to give help when needed, but as much responsibility as possible is given to the patients themselves.

CASE CONFERENCES

These are meetings at which the ward or unit team reviews a patient's progress and plans future treatment. Those present will include the patient, the nurses, the ward or unit doctor, the occupational therapist and the social worker. Sometimes the patient's relatives may be asked to come as well, and anyone else from outside the hospital who can help in the understanding of the patient's problems or the planning of his discharge.

HOSPITAL STAFF CONFERENCES

As we saw in Chapter Four the hospital team consists of nursing, medical and hospital administrative staff. If the members of this team understand each other's difficulties and work together as a whole their contribution to the therapeutic community will be much greater than if each group works on its own.

For this reason representatives of the three groups meet regularly to discuss how they can best promote the patients' recovery. New ideas are considered, old methods reviewed and each member has an opportunity to see what he can give for the good of the whole.

People present at these conferences might include, among others, the medical administrator and the hospital secretary, tutors, nursing officers, charge nurses, the catering staff, engineers, builders, psychologists, the chaplain, domestic staff, occupational therapists and social workers.

By making communications as open as possible and by trying to understand patients' behaviour the hospital team creates a community in which the patients come to see themselves as partners with the staff in their own treatment.

This is a difficult and lengthy task in which there are many setbacks. It is not easy for staff to accept patients as partners. Their authority is challenged. Traditional ways of looking at things have to be changed. New relationships must be tried out. Older staff sometimes feel that present-day methods are contrary to what they were taught in the past was essential for the patients' welfare. They may feel anxious and unsure.

This is why it is so important that the staff themselves should meet regularly to get to understand and trust each other. In this way they learn to support one another over difficulties and to appreciate each other's contribution to the patients' recovery.

PLANNED ACTIVITY

We used to think that nurses should 'look after' patients and 'do things' for them. Under this system they became dependent on the staff. The patient who always did as he was told and gave no trouble was said to be a good patient. The fact that, apart from doing what he was told, he often did nothing at all, was accepted as the inevitable result of his illness.

Today staff work all the time to make it possible for patients to do things for themselves.

It is harder, of course, to help someone to help himself than it is to do it for him. If mother is already behind with the housework and Tommy has put his jersey on back to front she feels very tempted to whip it off and put it right herself, but this will not help Tommy. Next time he will come with the jersey in his hand, expecting to have it put on for him. The same is true of making decisions and taking responsibility for one's own actions. The patients are encouraged to do anything they can for themselves, or for each other.

In his journey back to health the patient has to pass through stages which in some ways are similar to the landmarks on his road from childhood to maturity.

He learns to wash, dress and feed himself, to mix easily with his companions without fighting or being afraid of them, to take his share of the work of the world and to use his leisure creatively. It is in these areas of physical care, personal relationships, work and leisure that the hospital team try to build up his independence and personal responsibility.

Broadly speaking there are three groups of patients in the hospital—short-stay, long-stay and psycho-geriatric patients. The majority of patients admitted to hospital today will leave again in two or three months, and are spoken of as short-stay patients. Others, who may have to remain in hospital much longer, are known as long-stay patients. The third group is made up of people who have the symptoms of physical old age as well as those of mental illness. These are the psycho-geriatric patients.

SHORT-STAY PATIENTS

The main areas in which short-stay patients need rehabilitation are in personal relationships and in the creative use of leisure.

Ward meetings and patients' groups help them, and group projects, suggested and carried out by patients themselves, are encouraged, for example redecorating an old ward or building a rock garden.

Women may need help with budgeting the housekeeping money or with cooking and dressmaking.

Some patients, although they know how to wash, dress and feed themselves, may be too disturbed to do so and will need help in this area also.

LONG-STAY PATIENTS

Many long-stay patients have regressed to the stage of needing rehabilitation in all four areas. For them a detailed plan is necessary. It concentrates on toilet training, dressing and feeding, simple work and play and the renewing of contacts with friends and relatives.

Other long-stay patients are capable of looking after their own physical needs and are occupied in work of some kind, either in the hospital or outside, but have been in the hospital for so long that they have lost the wish to take up ordinary life again. They usually have their own social club and are helped by being encouraged to plan worthwhile leisure activities, particularly of a kind which will take them away from the hospital for a while, for example, shopping afternoons, visits to the cinema, or tea with relatives.

There are two types of work available to patients in most hospitals. The first is work in hospital departments, the kitchen, sewing room, library, laundry, gardens or staff residences. Patients who work in these departments receive pocket money each week. The second is sub-contract work sent into the hospital by local firms. The work varies from something quite simple like making cardboard boxes, to more complicated tasks such as assembling and painting toys and is carried out either in the wards or in a department specially fitted out for the purpose, called the industrial unit. Payment is made not according to the amount of work the patient turns out but according to the amount of effort he has put into it, and varies from 20p or so to a little over £1.00 a week.

Some hospitals have provided a third type of work by opening small factories in the hospital itself and producing goods which they sell to the local community. Payment here is in the region of £1.50 a week.

In addition a number of long-stay patients are able to

54

go out to work in the local district each day, returning to the hospital in the evening. Such work might include employment in canteens, shops, cinemas or factories. Wages are at full trade union level and these patients pay a certain amount to the hospital each week for their board and lodging.

Earning money is an important part of rehabilitation for long-stay patients. Many have forgotten the value of money and have lost the initiative needed to spend it. They are encouraged to spend pocket money, making their own choice of sweets, magazines, toilet articles, writing paper and so on. Larger sums are put into their hospital account in the finance officer's department, or into the Post Office Savings Bank, and drawn out as they want it.

PSYCHO-GERIATRIC PATIENTS

Because they have the disabilities of old age as well as a mental illness these patients need continual physical care. They can be helped by light work, games and hobbies which require little physical effort, but more than anything they need someone to sit and talk with them, to help them to talk to each other and to make them feel wanted.

Rehabilitation through work is called industrial therapy or work therapy. Rehabilitation through games or social activities is recreational therapy or social therapy, while occupational therapy is rehabilitation through the creative use of leisure.

Good occupational therapists include in their programmes what they call A.D.L.—*Activities of Daily Living*. It is not much help teaching a patient how to make a rug or a soft toy when he doesn't understand decimal money, has forgotten how to read a bus time-table, never notices that his shoes need repairing and can't sew on a button or cook a simple meal.

55

No patient, unless so physically infirm or mentally disturbed as to be incapable of helping himself, should be without work—purposeful work which will enable him to regain his independence. But quite a lot of patients who go out to work are lost when it comes to these ordinary activities of daily living.

A number of hospitals now have areas which are run by the patients themselves, as one would run a household. The patients budget, cater, cook, clean, make decisions about redecorating, furnishing and so on, in preparation for their return to normal life outside the hospital. Even long-stay patients can be rehabilitated in this way— perhaps not to the stage of returning to independence in the outside world, but certainly to a more useful, purposeful and interesting life within the hospital itself.

Rehabilitation includes responsibility for one's own medication, and most hospitals have now recognized that patients must be helped to become responsible for taking their own drugs, keeping them in a safe place and getting the prescription repeated. This means that it may be necessary for them to have access to a medicine cupboard key or to keep their tablets locked inside their own lockers or to take them to work, the nurses exercising only minimal control over the total drug situation.

Because there are so many necessary controls on drugs in hospitals, it is difficult for nurses to accept the idea of letting a patient handle his own drugs and when this policy is being carried out it is essential that the nurses and doctors should be in agreement and have complete confidence in each other. This is best achieved by full and frequent discussion of the subject, both during the planning stage and after the policy has been put into operation.

Ideally, all convalescent patients should spend some time in a ward where they can shop, cook and clean, with the minimum of help and supervision, before they are discharged to live in a hostel, or to go home. We might then see fewer people being readmitted to hospital because they could not cope with the ordinary activities of life outside.

These methods, together with rehabilitation in physical care when necessary, are used to build up a programme of activity for each patient, designed to restore his independence and personal responsibility. In addition the doctor will order whatever drugs or other individual treatment each patient may need.

The aim is to cure the patient if possible or to help him to live with his illness in such a way that his life is as satisfying as possible. This is rehabilitation and is achieved by planned activity in the setting of a therapeutic community.

6

The patient's day

Patients in a psychiatric hospital are usually grouped not according to what illness they have but according to the sort of care they need.

Some need physical care, others may want security and encouragement. Some must be rescued from a world of fantasy and all of them need a chance to try out new ways of dealing with their problems.

They have all come into hospital because life has become too much for them. The demands of society have been too hard and they have been unable to meet them. With many it is only a partial failure, but with others it is almost a total rejection of life itself.

One patient may be able to talk fairly easily with other people and share their interest in everyday affairs. He may be able to occupy himself in various ways and look after his personal needs, but his illness prevents him from carrying on his daily work.

Another may find that not only work but social contacts also are more than he can bear. It may be all he can do to wash and dress, eat his food and go to bed again.

Some patients are too confused, too occupied with their dream world, too apathetic or too depressed even to do this. They have regressed to a state which is very like that of a baby, completely dependent on other people for the basic necessities of life.

Just as one would plan a child's day according to his age and ability, so the patient's day in hospital is arranged to provide the kind of care he needs, to the degree in which he needs it. Hardly any two wards in a psychiatric hospital are run on exactly the same lines, except for meal times. These are usually constant, mainly because of the vast amount of extra work it would throw on the catering department if they were not so, but in most other respects the nurses adapt the day's routine to the patients' needs.

This is done to give the patient a chance to learn again, in safe and simple surroundings, how to meet the problems of everyday life.

The ward is a microcosm of ordinary society, as any group of people living together must be, but an infinitely variable one. Here it does not matter so much if he makes mistakes or behaves stupidly. The ward can adapt to him. He can be allowed to feel the effect of his behaviour, but only enough for him to see that this is not the best way. If he refuses to do his share of the work he may have to face the resentment and criticism of his fellow patients, but he will not get the sack, nor will his wife and children have to suffer. Meanwhile there is time to pause and help him find out why he refuses to work.

As he gets better he will move to other wards where the pattern is more complex, more nearly a copy of ordinary life, until he is finally ready to leave hospital altogether.

The layout of each ward is similar in principle. All will have dormitory space, a sitting-room and dining area, kitchen, nurses' office, doctors' clinics, bathrooms, wash rooms, sluices and lavatories, but details of furnishing will vary considerably.

In a ward where the patients can do little or nothing to help themselves the day will be very simple indeed, devoted primarily to keeping them fed, warm, clean and free from harm, and to giving them the feeling of being wanted. This is best done in a ward which is not too big.

The sleeping space may be divided in such a way that beds are in small groups, or it may consist of a number of small dormitories. A few single rooms are useful for patients who are noisy or restless at night and might disturb their companions if they slept in a dormitory. Some patients are frightened and confused by a large space or a number of people and for them too a single room may be best at times.

These patients, being unable to carry out even the most elementary care for themselves, will be incontinent, soiling furniture, floors and their clothes. Chairs should be upholstered in material which can be sponged clean easily and quickly. Floors and table tops should have a finish which does not stain and is quickly wiped over. The whole ward should be as bright and homelike as possible in spite of its simplicity. Colour can play a big part here and although a lot of ornaments are not necessary some pictures and a few plants can add much to the atmosphere of the ward.

These patients' clothes should be uncomplicated, easy to put on, warm and comfortable, pleasant to look at and easily washed. They will need enough of them to be able to change frequently. If they wear their own clothes it may be impossible to meet all these requirements. In this case it is better that they should wear clothes provided by the hospital and in this kind of ward they often do so, but the clothes should be issued individually to each patient and marked with his name. Each patient should have his own locker and his own personal toilet articles.

The main purpose of the day in this kind of ward is to bring the patient to the stage of controlling his bladder and bowels, washing, dressing and feeding himself properly and being able to make some contact with other people. This is best done if patients are divided into small groups and each group put in the care of one nurse, like a mother with her family.

The day consists of getting up, learning to wash and

dress, going to the lavatory at regular and frequent intervals, learning to feed oneself, a walk out of doors if possible, very simple recreation and going to bed again.

A strict timetable is laid down and everyone follows it to the letter every day. Ample time is allowed for each activity. There is no hurry. Constant repetition is needed and great patience. Someone doing up his own shoe laces, rubbing the soap on his flannel by himself, or going to the lavatory of his own accord are the highlights of the day. Even the smallest step forward is a source of pride for nurse and patient together and there is an affectionate bond between them.

From this ward we can pass on to one where the programme is more varied.

Patients are able to dress, wash and feed themselves, although for a number of reasons some of them may not do so. Some may be too preoccupied with their own thoughts to bother about washing, others are convinced that they are too wicked to be given food. They will need constant supervision and encouragement to help themselves.

The day's programme is still fixed by the staff and every period of the day is accounted for. Patients are not yet asked to make more than small decisions for themselves, but more activities are included in the day.

Nurses arrange for small groups of patients to help with the housework: some with tidying the dormitories, some with laying tables, washing up, dusting, or looking after flowers and plants. In doing this they work with the nurses and domestic staff, learning to share in the community life of the ward, to accept the discipline and the give and take which is necessary when people work together and depend on each other.

When the housework is done they will be occupied in other ways. Some will work in other departments of the hospital such as the main kitchen, the sewing room, the laundry or the gardens. Some will go to help with the housework in other wards. For many patients simple factory work is organized, such as making carrier bags, assembling ball-point pens or painting toys. At the end of the morning everyone meets for lunch in the ward, then off to work again for the afternoon.

Tea means the end of the working day and the beginning of recreation. The occupational therapists will supply the ward with materials for craft work and patients are encouraged to make such things as wickerwork trays and baskets, brightly coloured rugs, soft toys or leather goods. Small groups of patients may go shopping with a nurse. Relatives may take patients out to tea or for a walk. Sometimes larger groups go for a picnic or to the theatre. Later they may have a session of community singing, visit another ward for a game of cards, go to a dance in the recreation hall, watch television or have a games evening in their own ward.

Many of the patients in this kind of ward have been in hospital for some time and have lost the ability to adapt themselves to an ordinary working day. The programme here helps them to keep to a routine, to turn up in the right place at the right time, to work at the rate and with the accuracy required of them. It also helps them to get enjoyment from their leisure, to meet others socially and to make some contacts with the outside world. Yet everything is on a simple level and the nurses can easily modify the demands made on the patients to suit their growing ability.

The nurse in this kind of ward works with the patients all the time, she is a teacher and supervisor, a figure of benevolent authority but also a friend who shares their pleasures and difficulties alike.

Some patients will need to be more involved in the day-to-day running of the ward, particularly those who have only been ill for a short time. It may be that some of them are unable to accept authority, or fear to take any kind of responsibility. Perhaps they have always made other people decide things for them, or have been the kind of person who must always be the centre of attention.

Their need is for a situation in which they can try out various ways of solving their difficulties and appreciate the results without suffering the full effects of their mistakes. A situation in which, if they try to take responsibility and then panic, no great damage is done. They can talk over their failure with those concerned and try again. People whose attitude causes hostility in others can experience this without being completely crushed and can be helped to find more useful patterns of behaviour.

In this kind of ward patients will join with the nurses to implement the day's programme. For instance, each week the nurses may appoint one patient to be responsible for organizing the cleaning of the ward. It is then his job to get other patients into small groups to tidy the dormitories, dining-room or sitting-room. If they object or fall out among themselves he must attempt to resolve the difficulty himself, only calling on the nurse after he has tried and failed.

Evening entertainments will become the patients' responsibility. They may elect a small group who will arrange socials, whist drives, competitions, or musical evenings, the nurse helping with information, advice, equipment and anything else needed, but the patients taking as much responsibility as possible. Often this kind of ward will provide entertainment for patients from other wards who will be invited to join them for the evening. They may also send representatives to interward committees to organize such activities as a hospital dance, a tennis tournament or a talent contest.

Work and occupation during the day will be varied according to each person's individual needs and will be decided upon after discussion between the patient, the nurse and the doctor. Most of the patients will already have a trade or profession to which they will be returning when they leave hospital, so occupation will be directed towards such ends as encouraging self-confidence, perhaps by amateur dramatics, relieving tension by physical exercise, helping them to express their anxieties and fears through the medium of painting or modelling, and so on. Discussion of their problems with the doctors, nurses and other patients will also be helpful.

As he gets better there will be times when each patient can please himself about what he does. He will be allowed to spend an evening away from the hospital occasionally, to go for walks by himself, to shop, change his library book, or have tea out. At weekends he may go home to his family or to friends, sleeping away from the hospital for a night and then returning again.

In this situation the nurse is by no means a figure of authority. She is rather a rallying point for the patients in their efforts to find a way through their difficulties. She indicates the general direction, then stands on one side always ready with encouragement and support and alert to step in at once if necessary.

A few wards in each hospital will be run almost entirely by the patients themselves. A skeleton framework is of necessity imposed by meal times, doctors' interviews with patients and the general routine of other hospital departments, but within these limits patients organize the day's activities by agreement with each other. Generally these wards accommodate both men and women patients and the nursing staff is also mixed.

The role of the nurse in this kind of ward is often to be just simply another member of the group. This type of nursing, in which the relationship between the nurse and the patient is the most important factor, can in some ways demand more of a nurse than any other in the hospital because it requires her to understand and accept her own difficulties as well as those of the patients.

Her authority and her ability to help comes not from her position as a nurse but from what she is, as a person and from the relationships she can form with the patients. This is true of all psychiatric nursing, but it is more obvious here than in most other wards.

As she goes from ward to ward in her training a nurse may feel confused by the differences she finds unless she understands from the outset that the pattern of the patient's day is part—and an important part—of his treatment. Patients themselves rarely see this and unless the nurse has grasped it clearly she cannot answer with conviction when a patient says 'Why aren't I having any treatment nurse?'

When she goes into a ward for the first time a nurse should make herself familiar as soon as possible with the layout of the ward. She should know the total number of patients in the ward and any who require special care. She should then study the daily programme, comparing it with those followed in previous wards she has been in. The charge nurse and staff nurse will be glad to help her in this and she should satisfy herself that she understands the purpose of the routine and her own part in it.

7

Admitting patients

Going to hospital is a great step in the patient's life. It probably marks the climax of weeks of tension and anxiety. He has possibly feared for a long time that this would happen, but has pushed the thought on one side clinging desperately to the hope that it may not be necessary. He may have watched himself becoming more and more unable to cope and feared he was going mad. There is the embarrassment of the neighbours knowing, the feeling that he has let his family down, the worry over how they will get on while he is away, of what the people at work will think and whether they will really keep his job open for him.

His relatives too have been under strain. His behaviour may have been hard to understand. At first they may have thought he was just being difficult, perhaps putting it on. Gradually it dawned on them that something was wrong. Then came the long weeks of hoping that he would get over it. Perhaps visits to the outpatients' department and tablets to be taken. One day he seemed better, but the next he was just the same again. Was it their fault? What had they done? Why hadn't they noticed earlier?

Perhaps he has needed great persuasion before he would agree to come into hospital. His relatives are weary of the struggle, wondering still if they have done the right thing, ashamed of the thought that it will be such a relief to have him off their hands for a while.

Now, at last, he is here at the ward door. As he stands at the entrance to the ward he is full of doubts. Will he be shut in, will they let him see his family, will the doctors believe what he says, are the nurses cruel to patients?

From the moment a patient enters the grounds his hospital treatment has begun. One of the most important aspects of that treatment is the relationship between himself and the nursing staff. Right from the start he should be made to feel that the hospital is a place in which he will find understanding and help.

The nurse should go forward to meet the patient as he comes into the ward. This is more welcoming and less threatening than if she waits while he walks down the ward towards her. She should shake hands with him and his relatives and introduce herself by name. The normal social courtesies are reassuring and should not be hurried. If he seems reluctant to proceed, pause and give him time. It may be well worth while drawing a chair up and letting him sit down for a few minutes, even if it is in the middle of the corridor. A cup of tea can be helpful, and if it can be brought by another patient who can be introduced to him, so much the better.

Very often what patients need more than anything at this time is a chance just to look around—at the ward, at the other patients and perhaps most of all at you, the nurse. The fact that you sit down with him, that you smile and talk of ordinary things in a friendly, matter of fact way and are ready to give your full attention to him, will quieten some of his fears. He will begin to trust you, and this is the start of a good nurse-patient relationship. This trust is vital. It should be guarded and encouraged in every way possible.

His relatives have shared in his misgivings about coming into hospital and the nurse should not be sur-

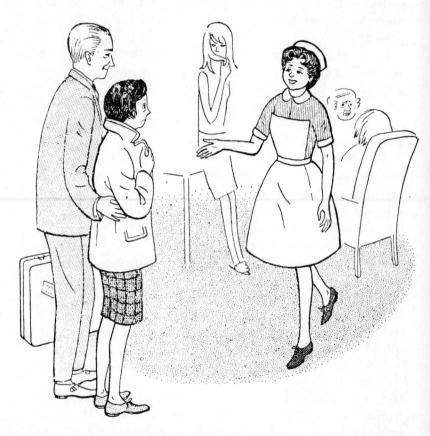

It is always hard for a newcomer to break into a well-established group, and the nurse should go forward to meet and welcome a new patient to her ward

prised if the relatives accompanying the patient seem rather difficult or demanding. When we are afraid or feel guilty we often take refuge in anger. Here again a friendly approach and a willingness to listen·and answer questions will reduce their apprehension. It is often a good plan to discuss the question of visiting hours, perhaps arranging the actual day and time when the relatives will come to see the patient. This gives' them a feeling of still being in touch. They will, after all, be able to see each other again.

The nurse, to whom the hospital is a familiar place, can easily fail to realize how exaggerated some of the patient's fears may be unless she makes a positive effort to use her imagination and put herself in his place.

Without letting them see that she is doing so, she should also be observing the patient and his relatives closely and later she will make a report of what she has noticed.

When the patient appears to be ready the nurse can show him where he will be sleeping. It is the practice in some wards to have patients in bed for a few days following admission. During this time they are allowed to get out of bed to wash and go to the lavatory and perhaps for meals also, but they wear their dressing-gown and slippers. This means that all nurses coming into the ward can see at a glance who has been recently admitted and should the patient wander out of the ward he is at once recognized. During the time the patient is in bed the nurses can observe him and get to know him, while he can get accustomed to a small part of the ward and a few other patients in the first instance before joining the full ward community. Many patients have neglected their physical health before admission and the doctor may consider a few days in bed to be beneficial for this reason also. This is not, however, done with all patients. The doctor may wish to avoid giving the patient the impression that there is anything physically wrong with him, or he may feel that the patient will easily adopt a too dependent attitude if put to bed. The nurse should find out what the doctor's instructions are before the patient arrives.

If the patient is to be asked to go to bed the reasons should be clearly explained to him and he should know approximately how long it will be before he gets dressed again.

The nurse may then offer to help the patient to unpack and put away the things he has brought with him. Some patients bring a great many more clothes with them than they need, and as storage space is usually limited this is an opportunity to discuss with the patient and his relatives which articles should be kept and which sent home again.

Rules about keeping small amounts of money, razors, matches, cigarette lighters, scissors and similar articles vary from ward to ward according to the patients' mental condition. In some wards where patients might injure themselves such articles are looked after by the nurses, but in others patients are allowed to keep them.

In every case medicines and tablets of all kinds are given to the ward sister. Valuables and large amounts of money should be sent home if possible. If not, they should be placed in a strong envelope, with the patient's full name, the name of the ward and a list of the contents on the outside. This envelope is taken either to the hospital secretary's department or to the principal nursing officer's department, according to the hospital's rules. A record is kept in the ward of all articles dealt with in this way.

The nurse will soon become accustomed to examining patients' property and will automatically know what articles can be kept in any particular ward. If she is not careful she will also very soon become quite insensitive to the patient's feelings about the matter.

Imagine having your own suitcase emptied by a customs officer—the feeling of resentment and helplessness and the sense of intrusion. This is how the patient feels.

He may have spent a long time deciding just what to bring and feels he needs everything in his case. The things the nurse is taking away are the very things he wants most if he is to keep up some kind of self-confidence and self-respect in the face of his difficulties. Now, it seems, he is not to be allowed to shave, he cannot keep his nails clean, have a smoke or buy a newspaper. The tablets which have helped him so much during the last few weeks are being confiscated, and the few things which have real sentimental value to him are to be taken away simply because they cost rather a lot of money.

The nurse needs to think about this and put herself in the patient's place before deciding how to act. One way is to sit down with the patient and his relatives before he opens his case and explain the matter quite frankly. Once his case is open the patient feels he needs to protect his possessions, but approached in this way, before he starts to unpack, he will probably agree quite readily with the nurse's suggestions.

Tell him that there are a few patients who might come to harm if they managed to get hold of the articles in question; that the responsibility for looking after patients rests with the nursing staff and for this reason they ask all patients to help by handing such things in for safe keeping. Explain that it is impossible to make exceptions to the rule and still be sure of safe-guarding the few, but that he will be able to have his things out to use whenever he needs them. Let him know that the doctor will be coming to see him in a short while and that he will be able to tell him about the tablets he has been taking. Regarding valuables and large sums of money, it may be helpful to point out that a hospital is in many ways like a large hotel and it would be foolish to leave such property in a hotel bedroom.

The doctor or the social worker may wish to interview the relatives before they leave and the nurse should find out whether this is so before she lets them go.

When the relatives are finally ready to say goodbye the nurse should occupy herself at a little distance where she can still observe the patient without intruding on their leave-taking.

If the patient is to go to bed he may welcome the suggestion of a bath. Not because he is necessarily in need of one, although some patients who have been too depressed or withdrawn to attend to their personal hygiene may well be so, but because a warm bath is a relaxing, comforting experience and he will probably feel all the better for it. Put to him like this he will most likely agree and be quite willing for the nurse to help him.

In the warm, steamy atmosphere of the bathroom, with the soothing effect of hot water the patient may talk more easily than in the ward. The nurse should listen quietly, giving him plenty of time and letting him know that she is sincerely interested in everything he may wish to tell her. The more information the staff have about a patient the better they will be able to help him, and every additional piece of knowledge is of value. The patient for his part will feel easier at being able to speak of his troubles and the nurse's interest will further strengthen his trust and confidence in the staff.

While listening to what he tells her the nurse should also observe his physical condition carefully, noting particularly any scars, bruises, inflammation, discharge or other abnormality.

When the bath is over the nurse should make quite sure that the patient is comfortable in bed. A warm drink may be appreciated and if he is in a dormitory it will help him to feel more at ease if he can meet the patients who will be sleeping on either side of him. Many patients have not slept in a room with other people since childhood and the experience can be a real intrusion of privacy until they become accustomed to it.

Every patient on admission is physically examined by the doctor, who will also make an assessment of his mental state. The nurse should tell the patient that the doctor will be coming to have a talk with him and to give him a physical examination. She should see that he knows where the lavatory is and that his dressing-gown and slippers are to hand. If he is not going to bed straight away he can be brought into the sitting-room or day room to meet some of the other patients, but whether he is in bed or not every new patient should be constantly observed by the nurse until she is told that this is no longer necessary.

When a new patient is expected it is a good plan to let everyone know, so that when he does come they are expecting him and ready to welcome him. His place at meal times should be arranged before he comes and it is helpful if, when he first meets the others, he can be introduced to those who will share his table.

When one is a newcomer it always seems a little hard at first to break into a well-established group. We can all remember what going into a new class at school was like, or arriving for the first day at a new job. What are the rules? Who are the important people? What do they expect of me? A ward full of patients can become quite a tightly closed unit and the nurse should do all she can during the first few days to see that the new patient is helped to feel welcome and accepted by the others.

At the same time she should be observing him closely. Is he usually in the company of others or alone? Does he talk readily when someone speaks to him, or is his manner reserved and his answers brief, or does he perhaps behave as if he had not heard the other person at all?

Accurate observation is one of the most important skills of psychiatric nursing and is of great assistance to the doctor. To treat the patient effectively the doctor needs as much information about him as he can possibly get. His background, his childhood, his family and job, his social life, all his interests, his likes and dislikes, his attitudes towards other people, each new piece of knowledge adds a little more to the jigsaw and helps to build up the picture of the person he really is. The doctor will get some of his information from interviews with the patient, some will come from the social worker who visits his home, some from relatives who come to the hospital, some from other members of the hospital staff such as occupational therapists, but it is to the nursing staff, who are with the patient for twenty-four hours a day, that he will look for the major part.

NURSES' NOTES

The nurse who admits a patient prepares a careful record of her observations for the doctor, and she should add to these at frequent intervals as long as the patient remains in the ward. In this way each nurse comes to be responsible for making regular notes on a small group of patients. These Nurses' Notes are then read by the doctor, who will discuss them with the nurse from time to time.

Nurses' Notes made on admission might include such topics as:

Appearance (What did he look like?)	*Examples.* His expression—sad, smiling, vacant, frowning. His physical condition—hair, teeth, nails, any marks, scars, bruises. Was he clean or dirty. His clothes—torn and neglected, or in good repair, stained and soiled, or freshly laundered.
Behaviour (What did he do?)	*Examples.* Did he sit silently, with his head bowed, or was he on the edge of his seat all the time, twisting his hands and looking over his shoulder. Did he weep, or shout. Did he argue with his relatives, or agree with everything that was said. Did he seem friendly, anxious, frightened, hostile,

74

demonstrative, reserved, preoccupied, suspicious. Was his behaviour any different towards the nurses, his relatives, the other patients.

Conversation Try to record it in his own words as far as
(What did possible. How did he say it—quietly and
he say?) calmly, or in jerky half-finished sentences. Was it easy to follow, or did he talk in a difficult, involved way, so that you lost the sense of it.

When the patient has been in the ward for some time the Nurses' Notes should also include reports on:

Sleep How long does he sleep. Does he wake early or late. Is he restless. Does he have difficulty in getting off to sleep. Does he dream.

Food What is his appetite like. His likes and dislikes. How does he eat. Does he bolt his food or take food from others. Does he refuse food. Do you know why?

Occupation What are his interests. How does he behave
Social towards the others. Is he solitary. Is he
  activities confident and persevering or does he tire
Leisure easily and need constant encouragement.

When writing these notes the nurse should go through the topics in her mind and try to recall everything she has noticed about the patient under each heading. She should remember that what is needed is a record of facts —what the patient said, how he behaved, what he looked like. The nurse's opinions and the conclusions she draws from his behaviour can be misleading unless they are accompanied by a description of what actually happened.

'Mr A was not very sociable at the dance last night,' may well be the nurse's impression after watching Mr A who sat between two other patients for the first half of the evening without speaking, then took a tray of coffee round at her suggestion and was finally persuaded to get on to the floor for the last dance. But to the doctor, who knows that he has always found social occasions a nerve-racking experience, this could have read, 'Mr A made a great effort and was more sociable than usual at the dance last night.'

There are some phrases which should be avoided if possible because they have been used indiscriminately in the past and are now almost meaningless. They really give more information about the staff using them than about the patient. For example, 'Mr B is cooperative', has 'settled down well', is 'comfortable', or 'satisfactory', has had 'a good week'.

Unless backed by more detail these phrases are most likely to mean either that Mr B has 'given me no trouble', or that 'I have not noticed him lately'. In the same way, 'Mr B has been uncooperative', or 'attention seeking', can really mean that 'Mr B got under my feet and I feel irritated'. It is much more useful to describe in what way Mr B was cooperative, or what is it about his behaviour that makes you think he has settled down well.

One of the qualities a psychiatric nurse must develop is the ability to be detached when necessary. Reporting objectively requires a real effort on her part. She needs to be able to stand back and watch herself, as well as the patient, as if she were looking at two other people.

This does not mean, as so many people think, that she becomes cold or hard. It simply means that she becomes clear sighted, able to see more of the truth about the patient and about herself. The more we can find the truth and accept it, the more use we shall be to the patients.

DAY AND NIGHT REPORTS

Other reports, which are made every day, are the ward day and night reports. These are not intended to give the doctor a detailed picture of the patient's progress. Their main purpose is to indicate to the nursing officers the needs of the ward in terms of nursing staff and to record significant changes for the information of all staff connected with the ward.

Each report should state the total number of patients in the ward, how many are out of the ward and for what reason, for example those on leave at the weekend, on pass for the evening, or out at work but returning later.

Patients requiring special attention should be mentioned, such as the excited patients, those with suicidal tendencies, or those who are physically ill. Newly admitted patients should be included with a note on their condition. If a patient has died, has been transferred to another ward or hospital, or has been discharged it should also be reported.

The night report will record the length and quality of the patients' sleep, those who had difficulty in getting to sleep and those who woke early, also any unusual happenings during the night. If a new patient has been admitted during the day the night nurse will make a point of visiting him frequently during the night and will report fully all that she observes. If he is wakeful he may be lonely or worried and she will do all she can to help him to sleep. She will also arrange to save a specimen of his urine on the first morning. Examination of the urine is part of the routine physical examination of every patient who comes into the hospital.

Patients, of course, expect reports to be written about them and most of them are quite aware that nurses do this. It is vital that nurses should regard all reports and all information about patients as completely confidential.

The patient trusts the nurse. Under no circumstances should the nurse break that trust. Few nurses would deliberately do so, but much harmful gossip can be started by someone overhearing a group of nurses laughing about the day's work as they go home on the bus. If you are ever in doubt ask yourself if you would like to hear someone you love spoken of in the same way.

The only safe rule is never to mention a patient's name outside the hospital, and the nurse must train herself to do this until it has become second nature.

8

Meal times, dress and personal hygiene

Washing, dressing and feeding ourselves are second nature to most of us. We do not have to think out how to use a toothbrush or whether the coat or the vest goes on first. We do these things quite automatically and when we have overslept or are late for work most of us can go through the whole process with quite amazing speed and dexterity. It is not until something goes wrong that we realize how complex these activities really are. When we are unable, through illness or old age, to do these things for ourselves we find how upsetting it can be to have to rely on other people to do them for us. Many people, even after serious illness, will say, 'It wasn't the operation that bothered me, it was not being able to look after myself'. Even a cut finger or a sprained wrist can make life tedious for a while and take away much of the pleasure of daily living.

Every mother knows only too well how much time and patience goes into training her children to wash properly, go to the lavatory, put their clothes on and feed themselves. As adults we take all this for granted and have forgotten how we learnt these skills, but at the time it meant a great deal to us. Learning was difficult. Some of our first conflicts were centred on feeding and toilet training, and although we are not conscious of it we have all been moulded to some extent by our experiences at that time and the relationships we formed with our parents who trained us.

Many patients in psychiatric hospitals are well able to wash, dress and feed themselves without assistance, given the necessary time and facilities, but others will need help. Under the strain of mental illness some patients are not able to look after themselves as they would if they were well. They may be too depressed or anxious to bother. Others may have strange ideas about food or clothes. Some have been ill for so long that they have forgotten what they learnt as children and are like toddlers needing to be taught all over again. Some are incapable of caring for themselves because they are too old or senile.

Helping patients to regain this ability is a most important part of psychiatric nursing for the following reasons.

1. The patient must be able to look after his physical needs before he can return to a full life outside the hospital.

2. Through helping the patient the nurse can learn a great deal about him. Every additional piece of information is valuable to doctors and nurses in hastening the patient's recovery.

3. Because bodily care is such an intimate matter the nurse who helps a patient willingly and with imagination can form a close relationship with him and can influence him in many ways. The relationship between the nurse and the patient plays a vital part in his treatment and this is one way of strengthening it.

The amount of help that patients need will vary from ward to ward, but the following outline of care and supervision will be applicable to the majority of patients. Care of special groups of patients will be discussed in later chapters.

PERSONAL HYGIENE

The nurse should see that wash rooms, bathrooms and lavatories, while properly ventilated, are kept as warm and comfortable as possible. Windows should be opened during the day but closed before bedtime; the nurse should also make sure that they are closed first thing in the morning before patients get up. There should be facilities for warming bath towels before use and drying them afterwards.

Many people are not accustomed to washing in front of others. They feel embarrassed if expected to do so and will, quite naturally, have only a superficial wash under such circumstances. While it is necessary for the nurse to be able to observe patients at all times, they should be given as much privacy as possible. Plastic curtains hung between wash basins and around showers will shield patients from each other while allowing the nurse easy access. A screen between two baths should be placed in such a way that each patient has an area of privacy but the nurse can see both at once.

WASHING AND SHAVING

Patients should be called in the morning in time to wash properly before breakfast and the nurse should see that such items as nail scissors and files are available. Shaving is best done with electric razors, but when safety razors are used one nurse should be responsible for issuing razor blades and collecting them after use.

Patients who may wish to injure themselves or to commit suicide can do a great deal of harm with a razor blade, and are therefore safer with electric razors. The rules regarding the use of safety razors and the observation of patients while shaving vary from ward to ward.

81

You should make yourself thoroughly familiar with the practice of the ward in which you are working.

BATHING

Everyone knows how pleasant a bath can be. The warm atmosphere, the soothing effect of the hot water, the freedom from clothes are all enjoyable. Tense muscles can relax, problems seem not quite so pressing, fears dwindle a little and we come out feeling comforted and refreshed. Patients feel like this too. Everything should be done to make bath time a leisurely procedure to be enjoyed by the patients. The nurse can help in this by planning the ward work to allow adequate time for bathing, and by resisting the temptation to fit the maximum number of baths into the shortest possible time.

While seeing that the patient has everything he needs the nurse should make a careful study of his physical condition. Does his hair need washing or cutting? Is he keeping his teeth clean? If not make a note to supervise this when he goes to bed and to arrange a hairdressing session as soon as possible.

Look carefully for any swellings, rashes, spots or inflamed areas on his body. Are his ankles puffy? Encourage him to pay attention to his toe nails and to the skin between his toes. Look for any raw areas of skin or white, moist patches which might indicate athlete's foot and report them at once as this condition is highly infectious. See that his toe nails are short and clean. If he has difficulty in cutting them a visit to the chiropodist will help. Notice if he has any trouble in getting in or out of the bath or in washing himself, and try to find out why.

Many patients will tell a nurse of their own accord if they are feeling physically ill, but others may be unable to do so because of their mental condition. The nurse should always be aware of this possibility and should watch closely for any signs of discomfort.

Patients should be encouraged to change their under-clothes at bath time and the nurse should be on the watch for signs of any discharge or bleeding. A record should be kept of menstrual periods and any irregular bleeding or missed periods should be reported. The first indication that a patient has piles may be blood-stained underclothing. Diarrhoea may also first be suspected because of soiled clothing, and again should be reported at once so that the cause may be found.

The nurse should train herself to make a detailed and methodical study of each patient in this way until it becomes habitual to her. With practice she will be able to do this unobtrusively as she assists the patient. At the same time she will be able to listen to anything the patient may wish to talk about to her, remembering that this is an excellent opportunity to show him that she is concerned about everything that affects his welfare, both physically and mentally.

When bathing is over and the patients are comfortable the nurse should go over all the points she has observed about each patient. Anything she has noticed for the first time and any change in his condition should be reported to the charge nurse and also written down in the Nurses' Notes on that patient. The Notes should include not only any physical change but also what he talked about and any alteration in his general behaviour.

WEIGHT

In most wards patients are weighed regularly and a persistent loss or increase should be reported. Variation in weight can be a sign either of physical illness or a change in the patient's mental condition.

BOWELS AND BLADDER

It is important to know whether the patient has his

bowels open regularly and passes urine normally. Again, many patients will be able to tell the nurse if this is so, but others may not. The nurse should notice how often the patient goes to the lavatory and if he has diarrhoea or frequency she should report the matter at once. Some forms of diarrhoea are highly infectious and can easily spread to other patients if not treated promptly. Frequent passing of urine may be due to kidney or bladder infection. It may also be caused by an enlarged prostate, a prolapsed uterus, pregnancy, or by anxiety and tension. Some patients may need reminding to use toilet paper or to flush the lavatory after use.

It should be made easy for patients to wash their hands after going to the lavatory and they should be helped to do so both by the nurse's attitude and her example.

HAIR AND COSMETICS

Most hospitals have a hairdressing salon and full use should be made of the facilities it offers. Regular haircuts add to a man's self-respect and a new hair style is a good tonic to most women. A hairdresser can usually visit the wards to attend patients who are unable to go to the salon, but when this is not possible a nurse can usually be found who has a little skill in hair cutting and styling.

In all matters of personal hygiene the nurse should not only be concerned that patients are clean and tidy, she should also show a personal interest in their appearance, looking for points to praise while helping them to improve where necessary.

The nurse who says 'Your hair looks a mess, Mrs Brown, I'll do it for you,' only confirms Mrs Brown in her feelings of inadequacy. If she can say, 'That's a nice frock, Mrs Brown, the colour suits you so well. May I help you with your hair?', she gives Mrs Brown enough encouragement over her frock to make her feel like taking the next step of doing something about her hair.

She also indicates that she and Mrs Brown will do it together, rather than suggesting that Mrs Brown sits passively while the nurse tidies her up.

This is important because everything a nurse and a patient can do together can be a means of strengthening the relationship between them and so drawing the patient back from his fantasy world to reality. What the patient and the nurse do is not as important as the fact that they are sharing the doing of it. The nurse should always be looking for ways in which she can draw the patient into sharing in activities with herself and other people.

CLOTHES

Clothes mean a great deal to all of us. Even people who say they don't care about clothes usually have their own favourite form of casual wear and would probably be annoyed if forced to wear anything else, so proving that they do in fact care quite a lot.

Clothes can be a means of expressing our personality or, like fancy dress, they can be a disguise or a way of changing the image we present to the world. Different clothes affect us in different ways. A man does not feel the same in a track suit as he does in a dinner jacket. A woman feels quite differently in a tweed skirt and a long evening dress, even her movements are different. The evening dress may have a full skirt but she will not stride out in it as she does in the tweed skirt. A nurse may feel that she puts her 'nurse' personality on with her uniform and takes it off again when she changes to go off duty.

Although most patients are able to dress themselves many do not care what they look like and their lack of interest is a measure of their illness. The nurse should do all she can to reawaken this interest.

No one can take pride in wearing clothes that have been rolled up in a bundle all night and are full of creases.

85

Every patient should have his own bedside locker and space for hanging clothes.

It should be possible for patients to send clothes to the laundry each week and the nurse should help them to do this. Some patients hide dirty clothes in odd corners or mix them up with clean ones. The nurse may need a lot of tact when getting these patients to sort out their things. If they are hurried they may become suspicious or hostile, feeling that the nurse is perhaps looking for something else, or resenting what they regard as interference. Much patience, courtesy and good humour are needed and it may be necessary to try more than once. If lockers are tidied and dirty clothes washed regularly there is less accumulation to deal with and a routine weekly turn out is a good plan.

Each ward should have facilities for washing small items which patients may not always want to send to the hospital laundry. A spin dryer and an iron will make it possible for them to deal with such things as shirts, blouses, socks and pants without the delay of waiting for the weekly laundry. Where these facilities are available it is easier for patients to maintain a good standard of personal hygiene. To be forced to wear a dirty shirt because your others are at the laundry and there is no means of washing this one overnight is enough to make anyone feel uncomfortable. If it happens frequently it can only add to depression and apathy.

Not only should the nurse encourage patients to keep their clothes clean, she should also help them to keep them in good repair. One afternoon a week can well be spent sewing on buttons and fasteners, brushing coats and skirts, going over collars and cuffs with a dry-cleaner, darning socks, mending shoulder-straps and generally smartening up. Done together, with the nurse, this can be much more enjoyable and less of a chore than if each patient works alone.

Ideally all patients should wear their own clothes.

With some patients, whose habits are poor, this may not always be possible, but when hospital clothes are issued to them the nurse should do what she can to let them have a personal issue of clothes marked with their names. There is little incentive to look after clothes if next time the laundry comes in you know you will not get the same ones back again.

Being made to wear institutional clothes is associated in most people's minds with orphanages or prisons. It means becoming a number and not a person. To the patient in a psychiatric hospital it can easily mean that he thinks he is no longer worth bothering about and he will retreat further into his illness. This is the exact opposite of everything the nurse is trying to achieve and she should do all she can to foster the patient's sense of being wanted, of being an individual who counts for something in his community.

Interest in personal appearance can be further increased by suggesting that patients might like to wear different clothes on different occasions. A dance or a concert, a visit to another ward for the evening, tea in the town, a country walk, can all be opportunities for a little thought about what to wear.

Clothes and general appearance are also useful topics of conversation. If the nurse starts a patient talking about present fashion trends, whether for men or women, she may learn for example something of his attitude towards the younger generation, perhaps to his own son or daughter. The price of clothes and the rate at which they wear out can lead to talk about money troubles or disputes between husband and wife. What to do with old clothes may reveal a variety of interests from gardening or rug making to bird watching or the Salvation Army.

The nurse who takes the trouble to listen to patients and is genuinely interested in their opinions can gather a great deal of information that will be of use to the rest of the ward team.

87

MEAL TIMES

We all enjoy eating and drinking. Meal times are something to which we look forward, and although none of us would come to any harm we should feel thoroughly put out if we had to miss our lunch or tea. If we are honest there are not many of us who feel real hunger before a meal. In the western half of the world almost all of us are too well fed for that. What we look forward to is the pleasant smell and taste of food and the chance to sit down and relax in congenial company. The housewife coming in after a busy morning's shopping really looks forward to that cup of coffee. Her husband, stopping off at the local on his way home, feels his pint is a just reward for the day's work and a pleasant prelude to the evening ahead. Many occasions have their own special food and drink—champagne for weddings, eggs for Easter or leeks for St David's day—while for some people a holiday can be completely spoilt if the food is poor.

In hospital meal times are just as important as they are in the world outside.

Plenty of time should be allowed for getting ready, eating and clearing away afterwards. There is often a tendency for meals to be rushed in hospital. Breakfast is hurried in order to get the ward cleaned and the patients off to their morning occupations. Lunch is rushed because the next shift is coming on. The time allowed for tea and supper may be cut short because of visitors or evening entertainments. Careful planning is needed to avoid this, but if nurses think ahead so that time is not wasted meal times can be pleasant occasions which contribute towards the patients' recovery.

The nurse should see that everything used during the meal is perfectly clean. Cutlery should be polished. No chipped or cracked china should be allowed to be used. Plastic cups, saucers, plates and tumblers are useful because they do not chip, but some plastics stain badly and need careful cleaning if they are to look inviting. If tablecloths are used they should always be fresh. A spotless table top is much nicer to eat from and more hygienic than a dirty tablecloth.

Whenever possible patients should help to lay tables. In some units they may also be able to share in buying the food and preparing it. Anything the patient can do like this helps him to come back into the world of ordinary people, away from the unreal world he has built for himself. The more everyday things he and the nurse can do together the better, and the nurse should be constantly looking for ways in which she can draw patients in to share in the day to day life of the ward.

The nurse should see that every patient helping to get the meal ready washes his hands before he starts. The other patients too should wash and tidy up before they come to eat and the nurse must see that they have time to do this.

Most patients will eat readily, but some will need special attention. Those who gulp their food down and might, therefore, choke, should be seated together so that a nurse can be with them. Some patients have poor table manners. Others may refuse to eat because they have delusions about food, perhaps believing that the food has been poisoned in order to kill them, or they may be so depressed that they think someone as wicked as they are can never deserve food. Any patient who persistently refuses food and needs much persuasion to make him eat should be fed apart from the others. The rest of the patients will not enjoy their meal if they see someone in distress about taking food.

As far as possible people who tend to irritate each other should be separated and friends should sit together. Small tables of four or six are better than large tables because it is easier for people to talk to each other across a small table.

The food itself is much more appetizing if it is offered in small portions and second helpings taken round later. Try to think of the things we all complain about in connection with a poor food service—cold plates, lukewarm food, an overloaded plate, gravy or sauce poured over everything when you never take gravy, splashes of food on the side of the plate—all the things that put you off your meal. Make a resolve that the food you serve will be appetizing in every way, with none of these faults.

If patients are capable of doing so let them help themselves to custard, sauce, butter, jam, paste, sugar, cake and so on. It may mean careful supervision to see that everyone has his fair share, but it is much better for the patients. When they are discharged people will expect them to be able to spread their own bread and butter and sugar their own tea.

When the meal is finished patients and nurse should clear away together. In many wards it is the practice for patients to be organized in a rota to help with handing round the food and clearing away afterwards.

Any occasion for a celebration should be welcomed. Anniversaries, birthdays, someone being discharged, success in a ward competition are all events which can be marked with just a little extra something. It need not be much. A choice of jams, chocolate biscuits instead of plain ones—it is the interest shown in that person as an individual which counts and helps him to feel wanted. Most catering staff are very willing to make a birthday cake if given a few days' notice and the nurse who is sufficiently interested to do so can easily give patients a happy surprise.

At weekends many patients are allowed to go home on pass, so that over Saturday and Sunday most wards have fewer patients than usual. Those who do remain are either not well enough to go on pass or have no one to whom they could go. Either way they are likely to be feeling somewhat despondent as they watch the others going off.

The good nurse will see here an opportunity to give extra attention to those who remain. There are fewer patients to attend to and the ward is generally not quite so busy as on a weekday. One way of putting the extra time to good use is to take a little longer over meals and make them slightly more informal. It may be possible for the nurses to join the patients for a cup of tea or coffee after the midday meal. At teatime the food might be laid on a trolley and some easy chairs drawn up to make a circle round the fire in wintertime, or taken out into the ward garden in the summer.

Not only is this a pleasant change for the patients, it shows them that the nurses consider they are worth spending time with. The tidiness and cleanliness of the ward must be maintained, but that sort of work should be fitted into the daily routine. The nurse who spends all her extra time cleaning out cupboards and ruling up books simply indicates to the patients that they are less important than cupboards and books.

9

Exercise, leisure and sleep

Many people who are mentally ill say they feel tired. They sleep badly at night and get up feeling tired. During the day because they are tired they feel disinclined to take any kind of exercise or join in any social activities. At night, partly because they have been sitting about all day, they again sleep badly. So a vicious circle is set up.

The nurse must help the patient to break through this circle on three fronts—exercise, leisure and sleep.

EXERCISE

Every patient should get out of doors at least once a day, unless the weather is so bad that this is out of the question.

The kind of exercise taken depends on the patient's physical and mental condition. Young, physically fit patients, who do not need too much supervision, can join in team games such as football, cricket or baseball with other wards. If a match can be arranged once a week the nurse may be able to arouse enough enthusiasm to get a group out practising for a while each day. Even if they are well enough to go out on their own they will feel encouraged if the nurse can go with them to join in the practice, and whenever possible she should do this.

Others may not be equal to playing in the team but

may enjoy watching and applauding from the sidelines. From these a supporters' group can be built up, which goes with the team on practice days to encourage and criticize. When the match day comes the supporters go with the team again to cheer and applaud.

The success of this kind of scheme depends on how much enthusiasm the nurse can rouse in the patients. The supporters' group is as important as the team itself and should be made to feel how much the team depends on them. If the nurse is keen the patients are much more likely to respond.

Quieter games, such as bowls or clock golf, are often available for less active patients, or simple ball games can be played in the ward garden.

Walking is the simplest form of exercise and is suitable for all patients. Those who need constant supervision can take short walks with the nurse in the shelter of the ward garden. Others can be taken on shopping expeditions and the most active may appreciate a country ramble if they are well enough.

Whatever form of exercise is chosen the following points should be kept in mind by the nurse.

1. Choose patients who are roughly of the same ability, physically and mentally.

Don't take an older patient with a group of active people whose pace may be too much for him. See that patients who are known to irritate each other go out in separate groups.

2. Plan the trip so that it is well within the abilities of all patients in the group.

For some patients who are physically or mentally frail fifteen minutes may be quite long enough, others may benefit from an hour or more, while some will be able to stay out for a whole afternoon. A short time, enjoyed by everyone and repeated frequently, does much more good than a long trip from which people return tired and dispirited.

3. If the group contains any patients who have suicidal tendencies, are likely to wander or to have fits, or whose behaviour is known to be unpredictable, extra nurses will be needed.

The number of nurses needed to accompany any group will depend entirely on the condition of the patients and where they are going. Twenty stable patients going to a sports meeting in the hospital grounds where other staff are present could be accompanied by one nurse who knows them well, while one acutely disturbed patient might need two nurses to look after him in the ward garden. In each case the sister or charge nurse will decide how many nurses are needed.

When two nurses go with a group one should be at the front and the other bringing up the rear. A nurse sent to give special attention to one or two patients should have them with her all the time and not allow herself to be diverted from them in any way, either by other patients or by nurses.

4. Allow time for patients to get ready.

Plan the outing in advance and tell patients well ahead of time. Few people like things sprung on them at the last moment. Encourage the patients to help in the planning.

5. Start the slow ones getting ready first.

Some people always take a long time to put their coats on and change their shoes. Get to know who they are, think ahead and see that these people do not keep the others waiting.

6. See that patients who will not go of their own accord are taken to the lavatory before starting out. Plan the route so that, if necessary, you can take patients to the lavatory on the way.

7. Check that everyone is suitably dressed.

Old people and those who move slowly must be warmly clad in bad weather. People playing games on muddy ground will need strong shoes. High heels will be uncomfortable on a country walk. Spectators may need overcoats but players will be happier in an extra pullover.

8. Tell sister or charge nurse where you are going, she will then know where to look if necessary.

9. Make sure you can recognize all the patients so that you can pick them out if they mingle with another group in the grounds.

Know how many patients you are taking and count them at every opportunity. Do this unobtrusively and frequently. Keep in mind the patients who need special attention and always know where they are. Practise this all the time and get into the habit of it. So that although you may be talking with one patient you are well aware of what the others are doing. If a patient wanders away and cannot be found in a few minutes return at once to the ward with the rest of the patients and report to sister.

10. Bring the patients in touch with everyday life as much as you can.

For example, if they are well enough to go part of the way by bus let them do so and let them pay their own fare. Before coming back stop and have a cup of tea and again let them pay for it themselves. Pay a visit to the Reading Room at the local library and have a look at the papers and magazines. In the hospital grounds stop and speak to other members of the staff—builders, gardeners, porters and so on. If sports equipment has to be collected take the patients with you to help.

11. When you get back see that outdoor clothes are put away tidily.

Wet coats should be dried and muddy shoes put on one side for cleaning. Some patients fill their pockets with all sorts of rubbish. Keep your eyes open for this and get rid of it tactfully.

12. Return in plenty of time for the next part of the day's programme.

You should have time to sit down with the patients

and talk for a little while about how the game went, or what happened on the walk, without having to rush off to some other task. In this way the enjoyment and benefit of the exercise is prolonged.

13. Report to sister or charge nurse on your return.

She will want to know all that you can tell her about the patients' behaviour. Any special incidents should also be written down in the Nurses' Notes.

A short time out of doors each day helps patients to sleep better and gives them an appetitie. At the same time it can bring them into touch with other people and stimulate their interest in .things outside themselves. Patients should be helped to feel like ordinary people as far as possible and nurses going with them outside the hospital should not wear uniform.

LEISURE

Most patients will be occupied during the day working in the ward, in the occupational therapy department, or in one of the other departments of the hospital, but the late afternoon and the evening are usually free for amusement and recreation.

There is generally an organized programme of entertainment each evening and patients should be encouraged to take part in the dances, brains trusts, concerts and other activities which are arranged.

These entertainments are helpful in bringing patients together, but not all patients can take part in them. Some, finding themselves in a large hall or a different ward, with a lot of new faces around, will feel too self-conscious and unsure to do anything but sit and watch the others. The nurse can do much to help these people by showing them how to use whatever leisure time is available in the ward during the day.

There is no need to organize anything complicated.

The simple things are usually the best because the patient is more likely to feel that he can join in. Whatever is done the important thing is that he should be taking part, not just passively watching.

Radio and television are in most wards now and many patients just sit idly in front of the set, not paying attention to what is going on. This does no good at all, but properly used radio and television can be a real asset in a ward by stimulating discussion. The nurse can study the day's programmes with the patients and together they can pick out something that looks interesting. It matters little what it is so long as the patients take part in the selection and, even more important, so long as they talk about it afterwards. A comedy sketch, a pop group, a record request, a story or a news item, each will provide something that the nurse can use to start an exchange of views.

The talk does not have to be on a high intellectual level. The clothes worn by the actors, the faces of the people in the audience, hair styles, memories of old songs we used to like, our favourite stories—these are things we can all talk about and most patients will have something to say if the nurse takes the lead.

Another useful tool is the daily newspaper. For example, one member of the group holds the paper and goes round the circle asking each person in turn to recall something he has read in it that day. The one with the paper checks each item mentioned and each person unable to remember something drops out until finally only the winner is left. This can be entertaining and it can also lead to quite a lot of discussion about the various items mentioned if the nurse steers the conversation a little. She can also mention the game earlier in the day and suggest that people get themselves well equipped with items by reading one of the newspapers.

Some patients will enjoy reading and the nurse can introduce them to the hospital library. A few may like to follow some particular line of study and here again the library will be of use. Through the occupational therapy department many discover talents, such as painting, modelling, poster design or carpentry, they were quite unaware of before coming into hospital. The nurse's interest will help them to learn more and to get the maximum benefit out of their new hobby.

Sometimes a group of patients can be persuaded to carry out a joint project, such as making and furnishing a doll's house or a farm yard. Scrapbooks sometimes appeal. For example, a scrapbook of all the Royal visits in the year, or one following the fortunes of a favourite football team. Schemes of this kind have the advantage that they bring patients into contact with other people, there is also the slight feeling of competition to see who can do most for the project, the effort required to collect and assemble the material, and the sense of achievement in completing something together.

Of all leisure activities perhaps the most helpful for patients is just talking, exchanging views, getting to know what other people think, considering someone else's opinion, having one's own ideas and prejudices questioned, gaining confidence to put one's own point forward, learning not to mind being laughed at just a little, even being able to change one's mind occasionally.

The nurse herself can make a big contribution here by being willing to share some of her own interests with the patients to start them talking.

Most nurses have some hobby, something they particularly like doing in their off-duty time. Half an hour could be set aside each week when the nurses would take it in turn to tell the patients about their own special interest, if possible bringing along something to show them.

As before, the presentation can be very simple. No one wants to give a formal lecture, or to listen to one, but talking about roses if you are a keen amateur gardener, or folk music if you have your own guitar is not all that difficult, and if the nurse is enthusiastic the patients' interest will be roused. Stamp collecting, holiday slides, making costume jewellery, model building, embroidery and making artificial flowers are only a few of the many subjects which can be found.

It doesn't matter that a talk on stamp collecting leads to someone mentioning a visit to France, someone else recalling war-time experiences and a third going back to the time when he used to collect butterflies as a boy. The object is not to teach patients how to collect stamps, but to draw them out of their isolation into contact with each other. To help them find pleasure once again in the endless fascination of everyday life.

SLEEP

If I lie awake for half an hour during the night it seems like an eternity. No one ever remembers falling asleep and the time when we are sleeping seems to pass in a flash. It is the time when we keep looking at the clock and turning over again that seems so long.

Most people are convinced that if they do not sleep at night their health will suffer. The less they sleep the more unwell they feel and this just confirms them in their fears. What is really making them feel ill is tension and anxiety.

Next time you are trying hard to go to sleep start at the top of your head and notice how many muscles you are using in the effort. To start with you are frowning—raise your eyebrows back to normal. The corners of your mouth are turned down—smile a little and you will feel your neck muscles relax as well. Your fingers are probably curled up so let them go loose. Just for a moment imagine that you are very heavy and that you have just fallen from a great height on to a bed of cotton wool. Feel how you sink down, down into the bed, as heavy as a load of sand. As your muscles relax you will get some

99

idea of how much energy we all put into our efforts to go to sleep. No wonder we find it so tiring.

People who are mentally ill often have difficulty in sleeping. The cause may be physical or mental, or both. It is the nurse's duty to find out if the patient is not sleeping and to do what she can to remove the cause.

If a patient says he has not slept do not argue with him. He is convinced, and the argument will only make him feel more distressed. Accept what he says and report it in the night report, together with your own observations. On the following night visit him every half hour and record carefully when he is asleep and when he is awake. This will help the doctor if he wishes to order a sedative for him.

Sedatives may be necessary at times, but there is much that can be done to help a patient to sleep other than giving him drugs, and a good night nurse does not turn to sedatives as the immediate answer.

The ward at night should be as quiet as you can make it. Doors which do not have to be locked should have a folded duster or similar piece of thick material, tied between the two handles so that the door cannot slam and make a noise as you go in and out. You should wear shoes which make no sound and learn to avoid all the squeaky floorboards. Remember that sounds carry and be especially careful when washing up or talking to other nurses outside the dormitory.

There should be enough light for the nurse to find her way about the ward but ward lights should be dimmed or shaded and no light should shine directly on to a patient's face. Be careful never to shine your torch into a patient's face.

The ward should be warm but not stuffy, and care should be taken to see that open windows do not cause a draught.

If these points are watched and patients are still wakeful the cause may be one of the following.

Physical
Unfamiliar surroundings
Uncomfortable bed
Feeling too hot
Feeling too cold
Need to go to the lavatory
Feeling hungry or thirsty
Hearing others snoring or
    coughing
Difficulty in breathing
Having a pain

Mental
Feeling anxious
Depressing thoughts
Bad dreams
Hearing voices
Feeling excited

A patient who has only just come into hospital may find it difficult to settle for the first few nights. Sleeping in a large dormitory can be very strange when one has been used to a small bedroom. All the shapes and sounds are different.

Bedclothes are frequently pulled too tightly across the foot of the bed. This can cause cold feet and occasionally cramp by restricting movement.

Snoring can often be stopped by turning the patient on his side, and someone who has difficulty in breathing will probably sleep more easily if his head and shoulders are raised a little with extra pillows.

If the patient is in pain you should let the nursing officer know at once. Some patients may not be able to say where the pain is or even to indicate that they do in fact feel any. The nurse should always bear this possibility in mind and if anything in the patient's behaviour leads her to suppose he might be suffering she should not hesitate to call the nursing officer.

Patients who are anxious have difficulty in getting off to sleep, while depressed patients sleep well for the first part of the night but wake in the small hours and cannot get off again. Many patients also have dreams which frighten them or cause them distress.

If a patient cannot sleep it is a good plan first of all to

suggest that he gets out of bed and goes to the lavatory. Then smooth out the bottom sheet on his bed, loosen the clothes at the foot and shake the pillows up. When he is in bed again fetch him a hot-water bottle, or a pair of bed socks for an old person, and make him a hot milk drink. Sit by his bed while he drinks it and let him take his time. Ask him why he cannot sleep and let him see by your attitude that you are concerned for him.

Often what he needs most is the reassurance that the nurse is there if he wants her. See that he is warm and comfortable after the drink and that he does not feel a draught. When you leave him tell him you will come back in ten minutes to see that he is comfortable and make sure that you keep your word. He will probably still be awake when you return because he wants to see if you meant it, but if you return in a further ten minutes the chances are that he will be sleeping.

Some nurses on night duty are inclined to think that they are out of touch, that there is nothing to be learnt at night time and little nursing to be done. Some get anxious if patients are wakeful and start pressing the doctor to order sedatives. Others complain in one breath that night duty is boring because there is nothing to do and in the next that they are hard done by if patients so much as open an eyelid before morning. Too often there is a lack of cooperation between day and night nurses.

This is a pity because the night nurse can be a most useful member of the ward team if both she and the day nurses realize how important her contribution can be.

Some patients find it easier to talk at night time. For one thing they have the nurse's undivided attention and for another there is the feeling that other patients and other members of the staff are not watching them as they talk.

The nurse herself has more time than during the day. However much she tries to avoid it there are times on day duty when talking with patients has to be curtailed because pressing jobs are waiting to be done, or because someone has interrupted. This doesn't happen at night. There is plenty of time to listen, to talk it over, and to write it down clearly for the doctor and the day staff.

If a patient is depressed or afraid it is much better that he should talk about it than lie there worrying. If his bed is in the dormitory and talking is likely to disturb the others, consider whether you cannot let him put his dressing-gown on and come into the day room with you for half an hour. If you do this remember not to get so absorbed in one patient that you forget the rest. Do rounds of the other patients as usual and keep your ears open in case someone else needs you too.

Restless, excited patients are more likely to relax if you sit quietly beside their beds for a little. There is no need for you to talk very much, it is your attitude which will communicate itself to them. If you are anxious and tell them to 'Hurry up and go to sleep!' it will do no good at all but if, having made them as comfortable as possible, you tell them calmly that it is time they went to sleep and that you are going to sit with them for a little until they do so, your presence will have the same soothing effect that a parent's can have on a fractious child.

Many patients look to their night nurses to give them confidence to face the night. They are glad to see the same nurse coming on duty each evening. If she is serene and gentle they draw comfort from her. Far from being boring night duty can be truly rewarding to a nurse who understands some of the possibilities of psychiatric nursing.

10

Helping short-stay patients

Many people who are suffering from a mild degree of
mental illness are treated in outpatient departments, day
hospitals, or night hospitals. Those whose illness cannot
be treated in this way are generally admitted to hospital.

This means that on admission most patients are
acutely ill. Some may seem at first glance to have little
wrong with them, others will clearly be quite out of
touch with what is going on. A few will be severely disturbed.

All psychiatric patients are at heart lonely, insecure
people. Many are also frightened, or weighed down with
feelings of guilt. The things they do and say are often
hard to understand and difficult to put up with. It will
help if you remember that behind the strange and tiresome behaviour is a likeable person, who needs all the
attention and help you can give him.

The first step then is to accept him, in your own mind,
just as he is. Don't make any judgements. Plenty of
people have done that in the past and it hasn't helped.
You may find his symptoms distressing, but be prepared
to like the person behind them. This is important. If you
can genuinely feel this way he will sense it in your voice
and manner and you will have made the first link with
him.

The second step is to realize that the more difficult a

104

patient is the more he needs your attention. Difficult behaviour is his way of asking for help. It is easy to give attention to the patient who responds with gratitude, but the patient who is coldly sarcastic to the nurses, the aggressive, overbearing patient, or the one who mutely resists every effort to bring him comfort, these are the ones we tend to avoid. The more we avoid them the more fixed their symptoms become and so a vicious circle is set up.

Most patients will have more than one symptom at a time. A hysterical patient may also be depressed. A suspicious patient can become excited. Patients with obsessional symptoms may be anxious as well. When and how you give them attention will depend on which symptoms are predominating.

ANXIOUS PATIENTS

Most patients are anxious at times. They worry about what will happen to them, whether they will 'go mad' or 'end up insane'. They wonder what is happening to the people at home, whether they did the right thing in coming into hospital, whether the doctor really understands what is wrong with them.

Some patients are anxious all the time. They feel that something dreadful is going to happen but they don't know what it is or what they should do to prevent it. They live in a state of fear which goes on night and day.

Because he is afraid this patient's muscles are always tense and the tension may lead to headaches, palpitations, a feeling that he cannot swallow or that he is suffocating and often to great fatigue. This convinces him that he has something seriously the matter with him, perhaps heart disease or cancer, and makes him even more anxious, which in turn increases his symptoms. He has no appetite and loses weight. He can't get off to sleep for worrying about himself and when he does drop off he has nightmares and wakes screaming. Sometimes he has panic attacks in which he feels he is going to die.

Most of us know what it is to feel anxious before some ordeal like an unpleasant interview or an examination—racing pulse, sweating hands and dry mouth, butterflies in the stomach and a frequent need to go to the lavatory. This, in a much more acute form, is what an anxious patient feels during a panic attack.

An anxious patient needs a good listener. It helps him if he can talk about his worries. If he has physical symptoms caused by his anxiety he will have been assured by the doctor that there is nothing physically wrong with him, but he will want to hear you say so too. Tell him how sensible he was to come into hospital and that his symptoms, although distressing, do not mean that he has some incurable disease. Be careful not to get so used to his list of complaints that you miss a new symptom when it appears for the first time. Report to sister at once if this happens. An anxious patient can have something really wrong with him physically, just as anyone else can.

At meal times serve him with small helpings and make them as attractive as possible. He needs tempting to eat. Find out from his friends and relatives if there is anything he particularly likes and get it for him if you can, or suggest they bring it in for him. It need not be anything expensive. His favourite brand of marmalade might be useful, or a tin of the bedtime drink he generally has at home.

Bedtime will be difficult for him. He dreads going to bed in case he will not be able to sleep, yet he dreads going to sleep for fear of what might happen if he did. Give him more of your attention in the evening. Try to see that he is not upset at that time. A warm bath and a hot drink might help him to settle for the night.

It may be difficult to spare enough time from your other duties to give to this patient. If so let him come with you and help whenever possible in what you are doing. He can talk at the same time and being with you helps him.

If he has a panic attack stop what you are doing and give him your full attention. It is no good telling him to pull himself together. You can see for yourself that he is sweating, trembling and gasping for breath. He feels he is going to die, but he will not do so. Sit quietly beside him. Sometimes putting your hand over his will help. Remain quite calm and keep your voice low. Tell him you are going to stay with him and that he will soon feel better. Your presence and your calmness will do more than anything else to soothe him.

As his symptoms subside he may welcome a cup of tea and perhaps something to eat. He will want to tell you

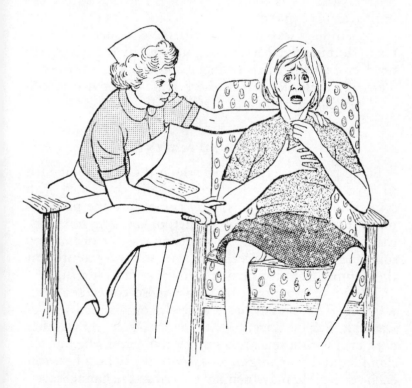

how he feels and you should make a careful report to charge nurse and in your Nurses' Notes about what he said and how he behaved during the attack.

If a panic attack takes place while his relatives are present they will be immensely helped by your demonstration of how to deal with the situation. They do not have your knowledge and are often terrified when they see him in this state.

When he is not having an attack try to keep him occupied with something which does not take too long to complete and will not demand too much concentration. Games are helpful because they relax him and bring him in touch with other people. Relaxation exercises in the physiotherapy department are sometimes ordered by his doctor. Walking is good because it is relaxing and it also improves his appetite.

Sometimes these patients will have a special fear of being shut in anywhere, or of going out of doors, and will need extra help when trying to overcome this. Special fears like these, for which there is no rational explanation, are called phobias.

OBSESSIONAL PATIENTS

Some patients have rituals which they feel compelled to carry out. These rituals are usually connected with some thought which constantly comes into the patient's mind. Examples are a fear of dirt, of catching some disease, of giving a disease to someone else, or of injuring someone he loves. He feels that the only way to prevent these things from happening is to carry out the ritual.

The most common rituals are those connected with washing. The patient has a special, complicated way of washing. For instance, he may have to start by washing each arm with seven strokes of the flannel, starting at the shoulder and touching the soap with the flannel between each stroke. He may then have to rinse the flannel seven times in the washbasin, rubbing soap on each side after each rinsing, before proceeding to the next part of the ritual. If he makes a mistake he has to start all over again and may even have to atone for the mistake by doing the whole thing several times.

He knows that his fears are unreasonable. He wishes he could stop behaving in this way but he feels compelled to go on for fear of some dreadful calamity if he should fail. In severe cases his behaviour may disrupt the whole of his life. He may spend so much time over his ritual that he cannot earn his living and may neglect to feed and clothe himself adequately.

It may help us to appreciate this patient's feelings if we recall the various ways in which we all try to ward off disaster by some magical means, or do things in a certain way for no more logical reason than that we feel better if we do them like that. Most of us as children have gone along touching every lamp-post or avoiding the cracks in the pavement. The housewife who likes the salt at the end of the shelf, then the tea, then the coffee and *then* the sugar—and not the other way round, please!—just likes it that way and will put it right at once if the jars get into the wrong order. A keen tennis player often has little rituals which he carries out before he serves. He may flip his racket over, or bounce the ball three times, or tap his foot on the ground. Many of us avoid the number thirteen. Although outwardly scoffing at superstition we would feel uneasy if forced to live at number thirteen.

In trying to help this patient the first thing to realize is that preventing him from carrying out his rituals only makes matters worse. If you do this he may become extremely agitated.

The most practical thing you can do is to help him carry out his rituals with as little distress as possible. Get to know, as clearly as you can, what it is he feels compelled to do and at what times he must do it. Try to see that at these times other patients do not disturb him so that he can complete the ritual first time without making a mistake. When he realizes that you understand and are trying to help he will feel he can relax a little and this in itself will make the rituals slightly less distressing for him.

The next thing is to keep him fully occupied. His doctor and the occupational therapist will probably have a talk with the nurses and arrange a programme for him which covers each hour of the day. Everyone should know this programme and help the patient to carry it out. The less time he has to sit and brood over his thoughts the better.

Eating may be difficult for him. Some obsessional patients have to be fed because they can never reach the point of decision at which they can take the food and feed themselves. Helping him to eat can be time consuming and it is essential that you should feel relaxed about it. This means arranging your work so that you will have the necessary time. If you are on edge to get on with something else he will sense your anxiety and become agitated and the meal will take twice as long. He will not be able to eat much so choose items which have good food value, and give him high calorie drinks such as Complan or egg in milk. Feed him away from the others so that neither he nor they are embarrassed by his difficulties. Sit facing him in a friendly way and give him your full attention. Try to cooperate as far as you can with his obsessions. After a little while you will be able to tell when he feels able to take the next mouthful and the two of you will work together.

It is often difficult to make contact with these patients because they are so intensely absorbed in their obsessions. Added to this it is natural to feel exasperated by their rituals. Yet they need approval and warmth. They are already full of guilt. This is why they are trying so hard to ward off retribution. When they see nurses and other patients put out by their behaviour they feel even more guilty, try harder to atone with more rituals, make more mistakes and feel still more guilty.

Do what you can to explain the obsessional patient's behaviour to other patients and to rouse their sympathy for him. Look for ways in which you can give him praise and show your understanding of his difficulties.

If you can bring him to trust you and at the same time work with the occupational therapist to see that he is kept as busy as possible his obsessions may become a little less severe. Meanwhile the doctor will be discussing his problems with him and through the combined efforts of the ward team he may gradually be drawn back into a more tolerable way of living, where his high standards and perseverance can be put to better use.

PATIENTS WITH HYSTERICAL SYMPTOMS

If we are to help patients with hysterical symptoms we must wholeheartedly accept the fact that they are not malingering.

The patient's symptoms serve to get him out of an unpleasant situation, to solve a conflict or to gain him some advantage, but he is completely unaware of this. The malingerer is perfectly aware of what he is doing.

It is important to get this clear because so often the causes of hysterical symptoms are transparently obvious to everyone except the patient.

If I say to myself 'My sister is much prettier than I am. I'll pretend to be blind then people will feel sorry for me and I shall get more attention than she does', then I am malingering. But if I wake up one morning truly unable to see, although there is nothing wrong with my eyes, then my blindness is hysterical and I do not know that it has happened because I am jealous of my sister, although this may be quite apparent to everyone else.

Hysterical symptoms can take many forms. The patient may complain of blindness or deafness, of paralysed limbs, of being unable to smell or taste things, or of loss of memory. A man may be impotent and a woman frigid. Sometimes patients have fits which are thought to be hysterical and when this happens you should take care to report the fits with great accuracy to help the doctor decide whether they are, in fact, hysterical or epileptic. In a hysterical fit the patient is usually unharmed by his fall, he is rarely incontinent, does not often bite his tongue, and the fit generally takes place in front of other people; but there are exceptions to all these points and accurate reporting is essential.

The patient's great need is for attention and affection. If he cannot get this in a legitimate way he may resort to coaxing, threatening, or to playing one member of the staff off against another. Often he will try to enlist the sympathy of the other patients against the staff. This is particularly easy for him to do if his symptom is, for instance, something like blindness or paralysis, which easily rouses people's sympathy.

His need for attention and affection must be met. At the same time you must show him that he can only expect attention if his behaviour is acceptable to other people.

The golden rule is to give him more and more attention as his behaviour improves and to withdraw your approval whenever it becomes unacceptable again.

Hysterical patients often have the ability to organize other people. Sometimes they have dramatic talent. You can make use of this by suggesting that he might like to get a group of patients to plan a ward entertainment. If he enjoys games he could be encouraged to arrange inter-ward matches and competitions. If there is a vote of thanks to be given at a ward function, or an announcement to be made at a social he might do this well. He could be a good master of ceremonies at a dance. These are all ways in which he can shine without having to resort to hysterical symptoms. Remember to show your approval plainly when he does these things well.

On the other hand some hysterical patients do not like the limelight. In this case try to reward him in some way when his behaviour improves. For instance, you might say, 'You've done well today Mr Smith. Would you like to help me get these prizes ready for the whist drive?' Be careful not to bribe him by saying 'Mr Smith, if I let you help me with the whist drive will you go to bed quietly afterwards?' The reward comes after the improvement, not before it, but you can encourage him by saying something like 'Why, that's fine Mr Smith! If you go on at this rate you'll be able to join us when we go to the cinema next Friday.' Then if his behaviour slips back you can say how sorry you are that you can't take him, but you hope he will be able to come next time.

The great mistake is to ignore a hysterical patient when he is not giving any trouble. It is tempting to do this because he can be irritating, but this kind of treatment only forces him into behaving hysterically in order to get attention. Be scrupulously fair with him. He must have no privileges that he has not earned. But at the same time be kind and let him know that you really care about his problems.

It is important also that he should get the same kind of treatment from each member of the ward team. In some ways he is like a child who will run from mother to father to get what he wants—'It isn't fair! Mummy lets me have it. Now you say I can't!'

It is helpful to discuss your feelings about him at staff meetings so that a common policy can be worked out. If everyone abides by this policy he will not be able to exploit the differences of opinion among the staff.

Finally, remember that if he complains of a new symptom it is not necessarily hysterical. Never ignore a complaint that has not been investigated. Report it to charge nurse at once. Hysterical patients can have lumbago or appendicitis, just like anyone else.

DEPRESSED PATIENTS

Depression is perhaps the easiest of all symptoms to understand. Which of us has not felt depressed at some time? In psychiatric patients depression can range from a mild listlessness to a depth of despair in which the patient feels the only escape is suicide.

Generally the depressed patient feels miserable and hopeless. He looks at his past life and sees nothing but failure. The future is empty. Life is not worth living. He will tell you everything is black. It is as if he were in a great fog or a nightmare. Often he feels he is guilty of some unpardonable sin and is unworthy of help. Because of his guilt he may believe that he is rotten inside, or that he has caused the death of millions of people and will soon be taken away for punishment (delusions). Sometimes he hears voices telling him so (hallucinations).

People who become severely depressed for the first time during the involutional period are often agitated. They may be always on the move walking about the ward, twisting their hands together, picking at their clothes, constantly repeating apprehensive phrases 'Oh dear! Oh dear! Oh dear!' 'No hope! No hope! No hope!' and so on.

Others are very slow in the way they speak, think and act. When you ask them a question it may be several minutes before they answer and when they do the words come slowly. This is called retardation. A few patients may be so retarded that they are unable to speak or move, or attend to their physical needs in any way. These patients are said to be in a stupor.

The depressed patient has little appetite and quickly loses weight. All his bodily functions are slowed down. He generally moves slowly, his circulation is poor and he feels cold. He often suffers from constipation. He sleeps badly and wakes early.

He will probably need encouragement over dressing. Left to himself he will not bother much about personal hygiene or about his appearance. But, as with all patients, a good appearance does help to restore his self-respect and you should help him to look his best. If he is retarded he will need to be started before the others if he is to be ready in time.

The stuporose patient will need all the care you would give to an unconscious patient—daily blanket bath, care of hair, eyes, nose, mouth, hands and feet, pressure areas, bowels and bladder. Artificial feeding may be necessary on rare occasions.

Although he may appear to be so the stuporose patient is not unconscious. He is just too sick at heart to utter a word or move hand or foot. He cannot answer but he can still hear what you say to him—and what you say about him, in his presence, to other people. Your attitude towards him, your kindness and sympathy, are even more important when he is so desperately ill. Try to talk to him, just very simply. Greet him when you go to attend him. Tell him quietly what you are going to do. When you have finished say that you hope you have been able to make him more comfortable and that you will come back later on. When you leave him say goodbye. Remember too that your hands can speak for you. Your gentleness when you clean his mouth and nose, the care with which you comb out the tangles in his hair, the firm support of your arm under his pillow as you raise his head, the friendly pressure of your hands as you draw the bedclothes round him before you leave, will all tell him of your continuing concern. When he gets better you may be humbled to learn how much it meant.

Meal times may be difficult for a depressed patient. He is probably not hungry and in any case he feels he ought not to have the food because he is so wicked. Often he thinks he must pay for the food and cannot do so. Sometimes he refuses to eat in an attempt to kill himself by starvation.

Because he eats little it is important that what he does eat should be as nourishing as possible, so choose his meals with this in mind. He easily becomes constipated so include as many helpings of fruit or vegetable as you can and persuade him to drink when possible.

If he is not too depressed he may feed himself with encouragement from you, but severely depressed patients generally need spoon-feeding. In this case feed him apart from the other patients. Make his tray really attractive. Serve food which is easily swallowed such as minced beef, eggs, milk pudding, sieved vegetables, stoned prunes, grated apples, pure orange juice, potatoes mashed with butter or milk. In fact a raw egg, beaten into a small helping of potatoes, mashed with butter and well seasoned, makes a nourishing meal which goes down with the minimum effort. It looks a bit insipid, so find a brightly coloured plate for it.

When feeding a depressed patient your attitude is important. It is no good arguing about his delusions, or trying to persuade him that he is not wicked. Sometimes a patient who feels he is unworthy of food can be persuaded to eat by pointing out that everyone who works for the community is entitled to his food and perhaps he would like to do something to help with the work of the ward in order to earn his meal. If this fails be kind, but let him see that you are quite determined that he is going to eat, that if he is thinking of suicide this particular way will not work, that you have ample time to spare and that the two of you are going to sit here until the meal is taken. When he has eaten he may try to make himself vomit. Be aware of this possibility and see that he has no opportunity to do so.

If you already have a good relationship with him and you are persistent in your efforts you will generally be successful. If you are not do not let it upset you. A patient who refuses food can present the psychiatric nurse with one of her biggest problems. Many people more experienced than you have had no more success. Talk it over with charge nurse and the other nurses. Compare what you do with what they do. Patients' reasons for refusing to eat may be complex and deep seated. We cannot hope to understand them all. It may well be that where you failed another nurse will be successful. The reason for this is much more likely to lie in the patient's illness than in your incompetence. Experienced nurses know this and will not blame you. What *is* wrong is to report that a patient has eaten when he has not. This is breaking trust with the patient.

Exercise is important for the depressed patient. He should be kept up and about and not allowed to lie on his bed all day. Take him out of doors when you can, but see that he is warmly clad.

Be careful how you draw him into the ward group. Nothing jars more unbearably than the professionally cheerful nurse who slaps him on the back and tells him to forget all about it and come and play bingo.

Remember there are ways of communicating with people other than by words. Give him your time and attention. It may be difficult to get any response from him at all, but if you can bring him just to sit in the same room with the others this is a start. Sit beside him when you can. Even if he doesn't answer when you speak he knows that you have chosen to be with him rather than any other patient. Putting your hand over his, or drawing his arm through yours as you sit or walk tells him of your concern. Use your eyes, your hands, your smile to show your sympathy.

Watch for the slightest sign of interest and follow it up. One day as you sit on the edge of the group you may notice that instead of looking down at his feet his eyes are following the movements of the other patients. Suggest moving to another seat a little nearer so that you can both see better.

He will be ready to help you before he is ready to mix with other patients because you have made a link with him, so give him something simple to do for you, like carrying a pile of pillowcases, or pushing a trolley. Encourage him to pay more attention to his appearance and compliment him when he does so. Show him how pleased you are when he can feed himself and join the others at meal times. Introduce him to a few of the more convalescent patients and encourage them to look after him.

SUICIDAL PATIENTS

Some patients are so deeply depressed that they feel driven to kill themselves as the only way out.

With the use of antidepressive drugs and electroconvulsive therapy, both of which are discussed in later chapters, this stage does not last long, but while the patient remains suicidal his life is in the hands of the nursing staff. Constant observation is necessary if he is to be prevented from carrying out his intentions. The nurses must know where he is and what he is doing throughout the twenty-four hours.

It is the practice in some hospitals to keep a suicidal patient in bed. He is not allowed the use of razor blades, penknives, matches, scissors or anything with which he might possibly harm himself. A nurse is always in the room with him and she does not take her attention off him for even a moment. When he has a bath, or goes to the lavatory, she goes with him and does not leave him, no matter how plausible his requests, until another nurse comes to take her place. His bed and bedside locker are stripped and searched once a day, while he is in the bath. This routine makes suicide practically impossible, but it also emphasizes the patient's isolation and may make him even more depressed than before.

It is now more usual to have a suicidal patient up and dressed and to encourage him to mix with others in the ward. If this method is to be successful every member of the ward team must be aware of the risk of suicide with this patient and a very high level of team work is called for. Someone must be within sight of him and aware of what he is doing at every minute of the day. Just how this is arranged will depend on the number of staff available and the daily routine for the ward. If there is a suicidal patient in the ward you should make certain that you understand in every detail what is required of you and then carry it out to the letter.

Never think that because the patient does not look particularly miserable the doctor must be mistaken. Some people can be deeply depressed and yet still manage to hide their feelings to a large extent. Never ignore a threat or a hint of suicide. The patient may have made the same threat many times before and you may have good reason to think that he is behaving in an hysterical way. Nevertheless, report the situation immediately to sister and stay with that patient until you are told that it is no longer necessary. Some hysterical patients do attempt suicide, and in any case this behaviour is a plea for help of some kind and should be treated as such.

There is no reason to be afraid of talking to a patient about his suicidal intentions. It may help him to sort out his feelings. If he complains that all the staff are watching him explain quite simply that you know he is depressed and you feel he may be thinking of suicide, but that you are so sure the hospital can help him, if he will only wait a little, that you are all determined not to let him carry out his intentions. The knowledge that the whole of the ward team is concerned for him will help to support him through the worst of his depression until drugs and electroconvulsive treatment begin to take effect.

In judging the progress of a depressed patient his doctor will look to the Nurses' Notes for information on any changes in behaviour and for reports on what the patient has been saying. Report frequently and think each time of what changes you have noticed since your last report—changes in how he looks, what he does and what he says. Has he shown any interest in his appearance yet? Has he started to feed himself? Is his weight rising? Does he still wake in the small hours? Is he less tired? Does he make any attempt to join in the ward activities? Has he spoken of his own accord to another patient yet? What did he say? Does he talk of anything other than his own unworthiness?

A severely depressed patient may be intensely suicidal but lack the physical energy to carry out his wishes. The first signs of recovery mark a danger point because not only does he still intend to kill himself, but he now has the strength to do it. This is particularly true of retarded or stuporose patients and your observation should be even more acute during the time when you can see that the patient is recovering but his doctor has not yet said that the risk of suicide is over.

Fortunately most depressed patients respond well to treatment. In fact recovery is often dramatic and the patient's relief brings pleasure to the whole ward.

EXCITED PATIENTS

People who know nothing about mental illness sometimes think, even today, that psychiatric patients go about with straws in their hair, screaming and attacking other people. In fact violent behaviour is extremely rare, but you will occasionally meet a patient who behaves in an excited way. A few of these patients may be suffering from mania, in which case their behaviour is said to be *manic*, but with the majority of them the cause of their excitement will probably be schizophrenia or drug intoxication.

An excited patient is constantly on the move. He walks about talking incessantly. It is difficult to follow what he says because he flies from one topic to another. He

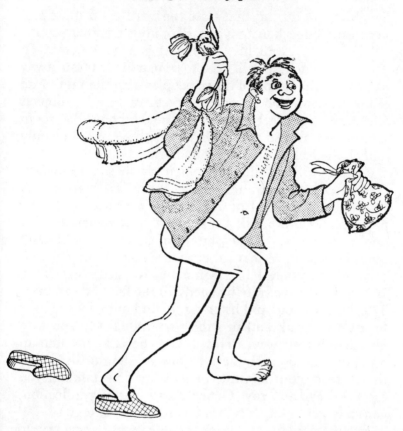

is full of energy and confidence. He has no time to listen
to what you are saying, no time to eat or drink, no time to
sleep, no time to go to the lavatory. He must talk, talk,
talk and keep on moving all the time. He dislikes the restriction of clothes and often takes them off. His language
is colourful and sometimes obscene. He often has bizarre
delusions and hallucinations, and as a result he may be
intensely suspicious and hostile. So long as he is not prevented from doing what he wants to do he appears to be
on top of the world, but as soon as he thinks someone is
interfering he becomes angry and aggressive.

With modern drugs his excitement can be reduced in a

few days, but during that time the ward team must prevent him from exhausting himself or injuring other people.

The more restful his surroundings are the better. In acute excitement he will need to be in a single room, away from the stimulation of other people, with the minimum of furniture and no ornaments, pictures, or other objects which he might feel tempted to throw about. The room should be warm so that if he prefers to be naked or only half clothed he will come to no harm.

Feeding will be a major problem. He has no time to sit down and eat an ordinary meal, but if food is given in a form that he can eat on the run he may accept it. Use paper plates and plastic beakers. Offer sandwiches, cake, apples, bananas, biscuits, hunks of cheese. If he doesn't take them at once leave them within reach and he will probably eat them later. Don't stick to fixed meal times. In this overactive state he needs all the food he can take. Try, by watching and listening, to find out what he likes to eat and drink and provide that. When you speak to him match your ways to his. It is no good asking him an ordinary question. He hasn't time to listen to the end of the sentence. But if, while he is eating and talking, you catch his eye and say 'Coffee'? with a rising inflection, you may get an equally brief word of agreement.

Excited patients are quick to sense people's reaction to them. When such a patient is in a good mood it is all too easy to be carried away by his boisterous high spirits and his witty remarks about other people. His behaviour has the dazzle of a firework display, but like a firework he can be destructive if handled carelessly. He quickly senses which nurse looks on him as a music hall turn and which one really wants to help him. His mood can change rapidly and his behaviour is often quite unpredictable.

To be successful in nursing him you will need to be calm, matter of fact, completely unshockable and have the imagination to understand some of the doubts and fears behind his excitement.

While he is acutely excited don't talk to him unless it is necessary. The less stimulation he has of any kind the better. Pay attention to him. Watch and listen closely. Let him have as much freedom as you can and when you need to stop him do it not by forbidding that activity but by suggesting another. Fortunately he is highly distractable. Just a simple remark from you can set him off on another track at once. Often words are not necessary. Picking up, say, a newspaper or a magazine will draw his attention away from what he is doing and on to something new. Sit quietly with him. Let him get used to you. Smile when he is amusing, but don't roar with laughter and never laugh at him, only with him. Avoid talking with other staff as if he were a performing animal— 'Isn't he marvellous! Just look what he's doing now! Have you ever seen anything like it?'

If he comes to trust you it will be less difficult for you to see that he gets enough food and sleep and to help him with his toilet. Once he feels you are with him you will be able to get quite a lot done by suggestion. Hold his dressing-gown open for him and he will slip his arms in without stopping in his flow of talk. Gather his towel and soap and make for the door and he will run beside you. On your way to the bathroom open the door of the lavatory and if you have gauged the time rightly he will be in and out again without demur and all will be well. A warm bath may help him to settle for the night, but you will be wise to wear a waterproof apron while helping him. When you come back to his room turn the bedclothes back and sit on the edge of the bed. As likely as not he will sit beside you. Get up and raise the bedclothes and it is probable that he will do the natural thing by swinging his legs up and sitting up in bed. Although still talking brightly he may be relaxed enough to play a game of cards with you and by degrees you will be able to settle him for a short sleep.

Fortunately he is not likely to remain in this acute stage

for long. When his excitement has been reduced he will be able to mix with some of the other patients but his behaviour may be extremely irritating or frightening to them. You will have to be on the watch all the time to anticipate quarrels or disagreements and to divert his attention before they happen.

When he is aggressive towards you do not take it personally. Some excited patients think they are very important people, such as the Queen, the Prime Minister, and so on. (These are delusions of grandeur.) He may think you have ignored his importance. Perhaps you remind him of someone he disliked or feared in the past. It may be that you have had to stop him from doing something. Whatever his reasons his aggression is part of his illness and is not directed against you as yourself. The best thing is to remain calm and deal with it as quickly as possible.

If his aggression is verbal say you are sorry that he feels like this and that you had no intention of upsetting him. Having said that much waste no more time over argument but try to divert his attention to something else.

If his actions become aggressive and it is necessary to restrain him physically, call for assistance. Never attempt to restrain an excited patient by yourself. Whatever he is trying to do it will only make matters worse if you tackle him single-handed and are put out of action yourself. There will then be no one to help him or the other patients.

If he is fighting with another patient and you wish to separate them, go behind him and put your arms round his waist. Your colleague does the same with the other patient and you can then draw them apart.

To restrain one patient a blanket is useful. Approach the patient from opposite sides with the blanket open between you. Wrap him in the blanket by yourselves walking swiftly round him, making sure that you hold the blanket high enough to get his arms inside. He is now wrapped in a cocoon and can be carried to his room with the minimum of disturbance. Once there lay him on his bed and control his movements by pressure on his shoulder and hip joints.

Never put pressure of any kind on his chest or abdomen and do not hold the middle of his arms or legs. These methods may easily cause injury, but pressure on the big joints at shoulders, hips, elbows and knees will control his movements safely. Have a fold of clothing or bed-clothes between your hand and the patient's skin to avoid bruising him. Relax your pressure as soon as you can, while remaining ready to reapply it at once if necessary.

Remember that the patient is almost certain to mis-interpret what you are doing. He will think he is being assaulted, that his enemies have come to take him away, that he is to be executed or tortured. Naturally he will be terrified and will redouble his efforts to get away. Explain —again and again. Tell him what is happening, even if you have to do it while you restrain him, and go on tell-ing him continually. Keep your voice low. Try to relax and speak gently, even while you have to struggle with him. Tell him you only want him to come quietly to his room and talk with you and that you will release him as soon as he stops struggling. Prove it by relaxing your grip, only reapplying it if his struggles continue.

In this situation, as in all others where patients are concerned, your attitude is vital. If you are angry your anger is communicated to the patient, through your muttered comments to your colleagues, by the expression on your face, by the grip of your hands and the way you move the patient. He reacts with fear and protest and the disturbance is prolonged. If you are calm and relaxed this too is communicated. You can anticipate events, in-stead of being caught unawares, as is likely if you are angry. Your words are more likely to reach the patient and calm him too, so that the situation is brought under control in the shortest possible time.

After it is over talk about it to the rest of the staff. Try to find out what caused the outburst and how it could have been prevented. It is a well known fact that where there is tension and disagreement among the staff in a ward the patients feel insecure and outbursts of aggression are more likely to happen than where the staff trust and understand each other. This is one reason why regular staff meetings are so important.

Patients suffering from manic-depressive illness who are only mildly overactive are said to be *hypomanic*. A hypomanic patient often lacks the dramatic quality of the manic patient and people's tempers are soon frayed by his constant chatter and interfering ways. He is well enough to mix with the rest of the ward, but he needs protection from their exasperation and they need a little respite from his attentions. If employment can be found for him he may make an energetic worker and get rid of much of his energy in this way, but he will need supervision. Occupations such as pottery or finger painting may help him. You may have to guide him in his choice of dress because, left to himself, he can put on quite unsuitable things. Women often wear hectic make-up. Substituting pale eye shadow and pink lipstick instead of scarlet may help.

WITHDRAWN PATIENTS

Some patients give the impression of having withdrawn into a world of their own. They seem to be indifferent to what goes on around them.

Left to himself such a patient chooses a corner of the ward, frequently by a radiator, and sits there silently for hours at a time. When he does speak it may be difficult to follow him. The words are plain but there seems to be no connection between one sentence and the next. Sometimes he stops in the middle of a sentence and then goes off on a different track altogether. You may see him smiling to himself, or making grimaces. Having sat silently for a long time he may suddenly get up and start shouting, or behaving in a peculiar way. He sometimes behaves in quite the opposite way to what one would expect, laughing over an unhappy incident, or being abusive to someone who is helping him.

Most people find such a patient more difficult to understand than those we have discussed so far. At times he seems to be living in quite a different world. He is often listening to voices and may have strange delusions about what he thinks is happening to him. Yet if we think of the everyday experiences we all have we may be able to understand him a little better.

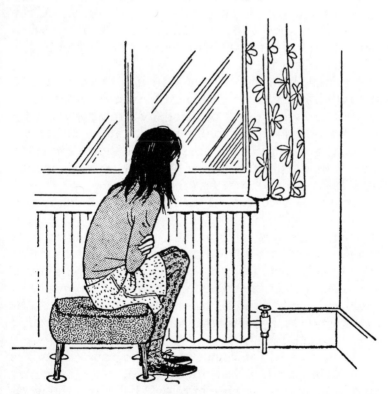

Suppose it is important that you get up at six o'clock one morning. You wake at five-thirty and look at the clock. Another half hour. Oh well, no hurry yet. Better not go to sleep though. Have to be out of the house by six-thirty. Mornings are getting lighter now. Seems to be fine. Funny how green the sea is. Must be because I'm high up. Floating like this you see a lot of the coastline. Better put those flat shoes on when I get up. Lot of walking to do. Strange, old Bob coming in like that. Haven't seen him since that holiday in Scotland. Wish he wouldn't keep just ahead of me. Can't seem to keep up with him. Better look at the clock I suppose. Oh—NO! It can't be! Not six-thirty!

You have been in and out of this world several times in the last hour with no awareness of the transition. At the time it all seemed to be one. It is possible that the withdrawn, hallucinated patient experiences something a little like this.

Although he appears to be oblivious of your interest the withdrawn patient is often quite aware of what is said in his hearing, even, as occasionally happens, when his withdrawal is so complete that he sinks into stupor. If this does happen he will need the same thoughtful care as the patient in a depressive stupor. When he recovers he may astonish you by what he can recall.

Because he is occupied with his voices or his unreal world he will need frequent prompting to wash, get dressed, eat, drink, go to the lavatory or take exercise. It is sometimes better to prompt him by your actions rather than by words because he may have a way of responding to spoken requests by doing the opposite. If you just hand him his flannel and towel he may walk over to the washbasin, whereas if you ask him to wash he may turn round and get back into bed.

When a patient does not respond to your efforts it is natural to pay him less attention and concentrate on those who give something in return, but this is the worst thing you can do for any patient. Those who do not respond are the ones who need your attention most of all and if you persist in trying to make contact you will gradually draw him back.

Make a point of speaking to him every time you go by, whether he takes any notice or not. Try to interest him in his appearance and compliment him whenever you can. Look all the time for things he can do normally and for any interest he may show in what is going on around him. You may discover that he can play the piano, or paint. If so encourage him all you can. These are both ways in which he can communicate without using words. Some mute patients will write if you give them pencil and paper. His paintings and writing may be helpful to his doctor and should be shown to him. It may be difficult to get him to mix with other patients at first, but perhaps he can join in simple ball games where the movements are repetitive.

Remember that his behaviour is unpredictable. It is difficult to foresee what he will do, so always be aware of him although you may be attending to others, and do not let him wander away by himself.

Since he cannot communicate easily it is important to look for even the smallest clues to his state of mind and you should report carefully any change in his behaviour or any response you get from him. Watch him when television is on and notice what takes his attention. If you see him listening to the other patients find out what they were talking about.

Find some time each day to sit beside him or to walk with him. Get him to help you in small ways if you can, to hold things for you or to help you carry something. Help him to use his five senses. Get him to smell the flowers you are arranging together. Draw his attention to the shine on the table as he dusts it with you and the pleasant feel of the sheets as he helps you put the clean linen out. The first time he reaches for his own knife and fork instead of waiting for you to pick them up and put them in his hands is a step forward. Let him see that you notice it and are pleased. All the ordinary little things that belong to this world can help to draw him back to reality if you use your imagination and do not become discouraged.

SUSPICIOUS PATIENTS

Some of the patients you meet will be convinced that people are plotting against them. It may be that they think they are being poisoned, or that the nurses and doctors are really prison guards in disguise who are only waiting for the right opportunity to take them off for interrogation.

The suspicious patient often thinks that every incident refers in some special way to him. Any little variation in the ward routine he feels signifies some new development in the plot against him. When a visitor comes into the ward and speaks to charge nurse he is sure the conversation is about him. When the counterpanes are changed on Monday instead of Tuesday it is a sign to his enemies that the time is ripe, and so on. He may feel that he is being influenced in some strange way through the radio or television, through the hot-water system or by means of electricity or radiation.

A patient who is convinced that events refer in some special way to him is said to have ideas of reference. Patients who have ideas of reference and feel that others are plotting against them are described as being paranoid.

We have all come across the person in ordinary life who is convinced that everyone is against him. Nothing is ever right. If the dustman misses one house in the road it is certain to be his. The neighbours spread lies about him, the children deliberately shout loudest under his windows and the cats always choose his garden for their activities. On the whole a suspicious person is not a particularly likeable character. It is difficult to convince him that he is mistaken and anyone who tries to do so generally ends up feeling thoroughly frustrated. It is a little different, however, when it happens to ourselves.

You go out of a room and as you close the door the people inside burst out laughing. For a moment you wonder if they are laughing at you. Perhaps you are worried, or guilty about something and as you walk along the street you catch people looking at you. What is it? Do they KNOW? Perhaps they can tell just by looking at you! You begin to avoid meeting people's eyes. You even lay little traps in your conversation to see if they will give themselves away. Pull yourself together! For heaven's sake, of course they don't know—and even if they did! And yet . . . why did he turn round and stare after you like that?

If you have ever experienced anything like this you will know how easily one incident can seem to reinforce another and your doubts go round and round in monotonous frenzy like wolves in a cage.

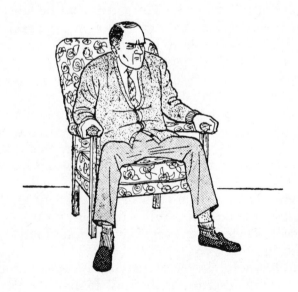

131

The suspicious patient finds it hard to trust anyone. Because he feels that people intend to harm him he may be aggressive and try to defend himself. In order to help him you will first have to understand as far as possible what it is that troubles him. Let him tell you in detail about his ideas and listen closely. Don't be drawn into agreeing with his delusions, just let him explain them to you. The more you understand the easier it will be to avoid alarming him and to anticipate what will make him aggressive. Some patients' delusions are marvellously detailed and coherent, others' are vague and changeable, but all the information you get can be used and should be reported accurately.

Frequently a suspicious patient believes he is being poisoned and meal times can be particularly trying for him. Arguing with him is useless. So is losing your temper. Accept that what he says is true for him and think of ways in which you can reassure him. It may help if you eat with him from the same plate. You take a piece and then he will do the same. Let him help you prepare a meal. As far as possible let him have what he fancies to eat. For instance, a boiled egg or fruit he can peel himself might be considered to be 'untouched by hand' and therefore safe. If he prefers to have his meals away from other people let him do so. Anything, within reason, that will calm his fears should be tried.

When he sees that you are trying to help him he may have confidence in you for a while, but this can easily change. One day you may be trusted more than anyone else, the next you are part of his delusions and in league with the rest. When this happens don't reject him as he rejects you. This only confirms all his suspicions. Another nurse may now be successful in helping him to eat and you should let her take over, but continue to give him attention in other ways.

He probably thinks people talk about him behind his back. Never stand near him and talk to someone else in a voice too low for him to hear. Either move right out of earshot, or deliberately raise your voices until he can hear clearly. Don't walk up behind him and say something to him. Approach him from the front, so that he sees you before you begin to speak. Avoid touching him unnecessarily. Suspicious patients often resent being touched and misinterpret people's intentions.

Explain to him what is going on in the ward. When another patient leaves the ward with a nurse it may be he is going to see the psychologist, or the hairdresser, or to have his exercises in the physiotherapy department, but to the paranoid patient THEY have got him at last and he is never coming back. Think of this whenever people come and go in the ward and tell him what is happening —again and again. Let other patients discuss where they have been, in his hearing. It is easy to find his delusions amusing at times and you may be tempted to laugh at him, but to do so would be very unkind and would undo all that you have been trying to build up.

The suspicious patient is naturally solitary and you may find he resists being drawn into the group activities. Start with something he can do by himself, gardening perhaps, then suggest that he helps you round the ward. After that he might be persuaded to join with another patient he trusts in some ward chores. You may get him to join a larger group by means of games such as tennis, quoits, or just throwing a ball from one to another, so that he is not jostled by others but can begin to make contact.

When they have just come into the hospital all patients are naturally very dependent on the ward team. At first they may be incapable of helping themselves and you will have to think and act for them in every way. But right from the day of admission you should start looking for ways in which you can encourage a patient to do things for himself.

This does not mean leaving him alone and expecting him to look after himself. It means being with him as much as you possibly can, encouraging him by showing your confidence in him, standing by and giving him time, not interfering, unobtrusively lending a hand when things get too much for him, but doing it in such a way that he is either unaware or can accept your help without losing face.

As they recover patients should take more and more responsibility. Convalescent patients can work in groups to receive patients transferred from other wards. They can decide where new patients shall sleep, introduce them to other patients and explain the ward routine to them. They can arrange their own work programme, suggesting projects and carrying them out with the help of the nurses and occupational therapists. Sometimes it is possible for them to plan their own menus, buying and cooking the food themselves. This is particularly helpful for women who have found the running of a home more than they could cope with. Problems concerning the management of the ward can be discussed at ward meetings and with the patients expected to help in working out a solution.

This does not mean that the ward team sits back and does nothing. On the contrary, they are all the time providing the background against which patients can try out their returning self-confidence and independence. Making satisfactory relationships with other people is always something a psychiatric patient finds difficult and many of the problems that arise are problems of relationships, either between patients or between patients and staff, or between the staff themselves.

In wards where regular ward meetings are held it is easier to give the right help at the right time because much more is known about the patients, and disturbed relationships can be discussed in an atmosphere of mutual support and trust.

Helping short-stay patients

Again and again people have found that disturbed behaviour among patients increases when there is tension and rivalry among the staff. When regular staff meetings are held it is possible to develop a real sharing between members of the ward team.

This is not an easy thing to do. It means being willing to discuss one's feelings frankly. For seniors it may mean accepting criticism from juniors. For inexperienced people it can mean having the courage to ask questions, to admit ignorance and to take advice. But those who persevere find that the incidence of disturbed behaviour in the ward falls significantly and less sedation is needed. A true community feeling develops, which hastens the patients' recovery and greatly increases the staff's satisfaction in their work.

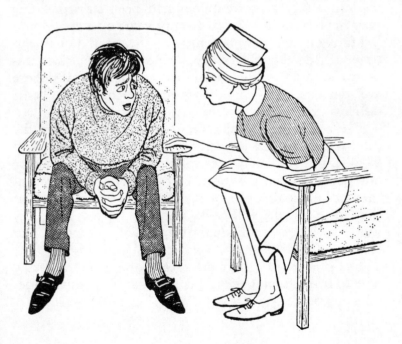

11

Caring for long-stay patients

REGRESSED PATIENTS

In most psychiatric hospitals there are a large number of patients who were admitted many years ago, before modern methods of treatment had been started. Some may have been in hospital twenty years or more.

Many of them have become incontinent and unable to dress or feed themselves. They sit about, silent and unoccupied, if left to their own devices. Occasionally there are outbursts of noisy, aggressive behaviour. These patients are usually spoken of as being regressed.

The rehabilitation of regressed patients is one of the most skilled nursing tasks in the hospital. They need help in all aspects of daily life—physical care, work, leisure and personal relationships. The difficulty is not only that they are incapable of looking after themselves, but that they have lost the will to do so. They behave as if they were no longer individual people with thoughts and feelings of their own.

The great skill in nursing these patients lies in being able to bring them back to life again as individual, independent people.

Physical care

The first aim is to teach them to go to the lavatory of their own accord and to wash and dress themselves.

Patients are usually divided into small groups, each group being in the charge of one nurse. The nurse works with the same group of patients each day so that she and the patients get to know one another. Generally eight patients is about as many as one nurse can help at a time and it may have to be less. Making the groups too large only delays progress and discourages the nurse and the patients.

Success in teaching physical care seems to lie, as with young children, in a simple routine constantly repeated, until the patient can carry it out for himself. Each ward will have its own way of doing this. You should make yourself thoroughly familiar with the ward routine for these patients and then carry it out exactly as it is laid down.

For example, a ward of around thirty patients might be divided into four groups. Every patient should have his own flannel, toothbrush and towel and his own bedside locker. Toilet accommodation in most hospitals is limited and some staggering is needed to avoid queues and over-crowding, so that first thing in the morning those in group one might get up and go to the lavatory while group two make beds. Group one could then wash and dress and return to make their beds while group two go to the lavatory, and so on. As soon as groups one and two are well started groups three and four can begin.

At first you will have to do everything for the patient. You will probably have to remind him to use toilet paper and to flush the lavatory after using it. But right from the start you should show him that you expect him to be able to do it for himself. Day after day you may say 'Rub the soap on the flannel. Now wash your face' without results, but the day will come when his hand reaches out. When this happens let him see how pleased you are. Tell the other patients, in his hearing, how well Mr A is getting on.

Remember that you are awakening the patient's individuality. Although it may be hard to arrange he should have as much privacy as possible when washing. Adults in ordinary life do not usually stand naked in a line in front of uncurtained wash basins, nor do they usually walk about unclothed in front of strangers. If the hospital has not yet been able to improve poor washroom facilities do what you can by placing screens so that patients are shielded from each other while your view of the group remains unhindered. Encourage them to use their dressing-gowns. You will have to watch that flannels and towels are not mixed up. Toothbrushes, flannels, combs and hairbrushes should be marked with the owner's name. They may get used for many purposes, so flannels should be boiled each evening and toothbrushes thoroughly washed in soapy water. Hairbrushes and combs will need washing frequently.

Dressing should be carried out in the same order every day, with the same promptings. Again, you may put the patient's vest in his hand and day after day he lets it fall to the floor, but one morning he will gather it up and try to draw it over his head—another achievement to be applauded and talked about. Tell the other nurses how pleased you are in a voice loud enough for him to hear.

Do not underestimate the effect of your own personal hygiene and your own appearance on the patient. Set him a high standard to aim at by being really well groomed yourself. Try not only to train him in routine bodily care but to reawaken the pleasure most people get out of washing and dressing. Talk about the flavours of different toothpastes, get him to smell the soap, remark how you enjoy a rub with a good rough towel, how pleasant it is to put on a clean shirt or blouse. Time after time you will get no response. It takes a good psychiatric nurse to reach a patient like this, but one day he will lift his head and look at you with the beginnings of a real smile.

Going to the lavatory, washing hands and tidying hair

and clothes is repeated every four hours, before the mid-day meal, before tea and before supper. No exceptions are made, no excuses allowed, but as with children the same routine is repeated again and again, until the patients can care for themselves.

The next step is to help them to feed themselves. Some patients may be quite unable to do this, some may eat but use their hands instead of the knife and fork, or throw food about, some may gobble their food and steal from their neighbours' plates, others may take food away to hide it.

Make sure that everyone has teeth to eat with. Let charge nurse know if a patient seems to have difficulty in biting food or if he needs dentures. See that patients who do have dentures are wearing them before the meal starts.

If a patient cannot feed himself tie a large bib round him to protect his clothes and start with a spoon, putting it in his hand and guiding it to his mouth. At this stage try to choose food which is easily managed in a spoon so that he does not make too much mess and feel conspicuous. As soon as he can use the spoon move on to a knife and fork.

If a patient has poor table manners, you need to decide whether he has, as it were, gone back to being a baby, grabbing at everything with both hands and playing with it, or whether he remembers how to eat but is just not bothering to use a knife and fork properly. If he has forgotten you will have to start teaching him with bib and spoon. If you feel he can feed properly when he wants to, make him want to by appealing to his need for approval. 'Why, Mr A, I thought you could do better than that. I was expecting you to set us an example!'

The patient who stuffs his mouth full and eats his neighbour's helping as well as his own, may possibly fear that his share will be taken away if he doesn't hurry, or that there is not enough to go round, or that this is the last meal before doomsday, and so on. Try to find out what worries him if you can and put it right. Serve small helpings of food and cut it into small pieces so that he doesn't choke himself. Sit him out of reach of other people's plates. Assure him that there is plenty now and more later on. As he finishes offer second and third helpings, until he has had all he wants.

The patient who takes food away and hides it may be trying to avoid eating altogether. If you think he is suspicious try eating with him from the same plate. If he is depressed be firm in feeding him and give him all the extra attention you can in between meal times. Let him see that you are interested in him and want him to get better. The quickest way to make a depressed person eat is to make him want to live. On the other hand the patient may eat at meal times and still take food away to hide. This may be because supper is too early for him and he gets hungry at night. Try giving him bread and butter at bedtime. If this doesn't work it may be that he hoards anything he can get hold of, including food. If so try interesting him in collecting something more useful such as cartoon strips to make a scrap book, or pictures from magazines to be used when cut-outs are needed.

Each group of patients should help with preparations for the meal. At first there may only be one or two who can do anything at all, but gradually you should lead them on to laying the tables, carrying the food, helping themselves to condiments, passing plates, helping to clear away and wash up afterwards.

Look for tiny ways in which they are improving and point them out, both to the patient himself and to other people.

Try to find little privileges and rewards which will encourage them. Only people who know how to keep their nails clean may help with laying tables. To help prepare the meal you must wash after going to the lavatory, without being told. To sit with the others at meal times you must be able to feed yourself. Those who can use a knife and fork sit at the top tables. When you can wash, dress and feed yourself unaided you may become a group leader and show others how to do it.

You know, in your own work in the ward, how a word of praise from sister can spur you on more than any amount of criticism. Remember this with the patients and praise them whenever you can.

While they are re-learning how to attend to their personal hygiene and feed themselves a start is also made in the fields of work, leisure and personal relationships.

It is of no use to have a clean, well fed patient if he spends the rest of the day sitting silently in a chair. Moreover it has been found that incontinence is often overcome more readily if patients are occupied and receiving attention during the rest of the day.

Work

At first work is very simple indeed and only takes up part of the day. The occupational therapists work closely with the nursing staff in helping to find tasks which are within the patients' abilities.

There may be old furniture in the ward which can be sanded and polished. Old bedsteads can be taken one at a time, rubbed down and enamelled. Cutlery and glasses need polishing. Plastic cups and saucers get stained and need regular scouring. Metal ash trays can be cleaned and painted with clear varnish. Old-fashioned picture frames can be modernized by rubbing down and painting with white enamel. Dining-room tables and chairs can be painted in bright colours.

The industrial unit may be able to provide simple work which can be done in the ward, such as folding greeting cards, or assembling gift boxes. Rug making and weaving may be introduced by the occupational therapists.

The work period has a fixed place in the ward timetable, usually in the morning. The timetable is pinned up on the ward noticeboard and you can help patients to be punctual by constantly referring to it and talking about the next item on the programme.

Work generally goes on for a couple of hours, with a break halfway through for a mid-morning drink so that the effort of concentrating is not too tiring.

Payment is important. It means that the patient is recognized as an individual, that he is worth something in the community. To be without money in a society largely built upon it can be demoralizing. It is practically impossible for an ordinary person to hold up his head and keep his self respect if he is consistently prevented from earning money. In times of mass unemployment some people come to look very much like regressed psychiatric patients.

The value of the work done is judged not by the length of the time the patient takes doing it, not by the quality of the finished product, but by the amount of effort he puts into it. Charge nurse, the other nurses and the occupational therapists will decide together how much each patient should receive at the end of the week. At first the amounts will only be a few pence, but as progress is made he will earn more. The increase in his earnings is tangible proof to him that he is becoming worth more, that he counts for something in his group, that people notice what he does and recognize the effort he makes.

Leisure

Once work is finished the rest of the day can be spent in leisure activities, such as the following.

Outdoor exercise. Regressed patients need exercise and fresh air and should be out of doors for some time each day if at all possible. At first they will go only into the ward garden, later into the hospital grounds and, when enough progress has been made, into the world outside.

Games can be played in the ward garden. Standing in a circle and throwing a ball to someone in the centre, hockey with walking sticks, quoits or tennis with an improvised net, rounders, under and over, or relay races all need the minimum of equipment and give enjoyable exercise.

Gardening may interest many patients. Each group can have a part of the garden and a date could be fixed for someone to award a prize to the best group. Patients can, of course, join together to choose and buy their own packets of seed and much pleasant discussion can go on about what to grow and how to lay out their particular plot to the best advantage. They can be encouraged to club together and buy a gardening magazine and to listen to gardening programmes on radio and television. Use can be made of their interest by letting it be known that as soon as a group is consistently neat and tidy in appearance they can be taken on a tour of the hospital

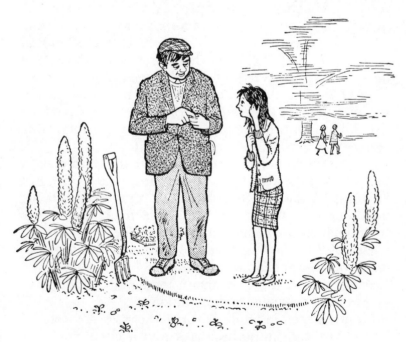

grounds to get some ideas. The head gardener can be approached and will probably be only too pleased to answer questions and give advice.

Walking is an excellent form of exercise. Patients should go in small groups so that the nurses can give them individual attention. A short distance, enjoyed by everyone, is much better than a long walk which some may find tiring. As you go along draw the patients' attention to everything around them. Some may not have been outside the ward for months and may have forgotten what it is like. Point out different parts of the hospital, the boiler house, the workshops, the social centre, the industrial unit and talk about the work that goes on there. Stop and look at trees, flowers, animals and name them all. Get the patients to start a collection of grasses or wild flowers, take them back to the ward, press them between newspaper and make a scrapbook. Suggest that they look for additions to the collection each time they go out. Get a book from the hospital library which will tell them the names of the grasses and flowers. Speak to as many people as you can on the walk. Outside the hospital look at what other people are doing, the postman, the milkman, people shopping or taking the children out. Remember, these patients are learning all over again what goes on in the world.

Whenever patients are going to leave the ward make a point of talking about personal appearance. Hair must be brushed, shoes polished, clothes neat and suitable, hands clean. Only those who have made themselves smart enough can come. Don't do it all for them. Use the pleasure of the outing as a way of stimulating them to improve their appearance themselves.

Indoor exercise. If the weather is too bad to go out try to arrange some form of exercise indoors.

Simple stretching and bending exercises are helpful. The chairs can be pushed back and a circle made for marching, or running. Arm swinging and neck exercises are relaxing and will improve posture. Turn on the radio or use a record player and exercise to music. Better still, get a patient to play the piano, or play it yourself. Musical chairs, oranges and lemons and simple square dancing all get people moving and enjoying themselves.

Shopping. If earning money increases a person's self-respect and independence, so does spending it.

Patients should be encouraged to spend a little of their money each week and save the rest. Even if they only earn three shillings some can be put aside for the future and some spent for today's needs. Saving should be presented to them as actively preparing for the time when they will be better and will want some money behind them. This indicates that there really is a future worth planning for. Help them to budget the amount available for spending now—sweets, cigarettes, a comb, writing paper, a paperback book, toilet articles—what should have priority this week?

Make full use of the hospital shop. Take patients a few at a time and, as before, insist on a good appearance. Anyone who has not bothered to smarten up will have to wait until next week. On the way talk about the places you pass, other wards, the main kitchen, the laundry, the stores. Greet as many people as you can and encourage patients to do so too. At the shop introduce them to the person behind the counter and on subsequent visits recall his name to them before you get to the shop, so that they can use it when speaking to him.

Once there let them take their time and make their own choice, only intervening if a patient really needs help. Back in the ward, talk over what has been bought and help patients to mark the articles with their names when necessary.

Grooming. In addition to the daily routine of washing and dressing, time should be made in the ward programme every week for a general grooming session.

Clothes can be turned out and inspected for snags, lost buttons, food stains, greasy collars and so on. Stockings can be mended, small items washed, trousers pressed, shoes polished.

Find a suitable box and make a grooming kit. Ask the patients what should go into it—darning needles, sock wool, coloured cottons, sewing needles, thimbles, scissors, elastic, shirt buttons, dry cleaner, a stiff brush for tweeds and a softer one for woollens. Help them to paint it or cover it in some way. Have a group looking through magazines for suitable pictures to cut out and use in decorating it.

Hair, skin and nails need attention too. Men should go regularly to have their hair cut. Women can be interested in trying out different styles on each other in the ward. All patients can benefit from a manicure session. Encourage women to use a few cosmetics. Get some lipsticks in various shades and let them see the effect on each other. Next time you go to the hospital shop draw their attention to the pretty little cosmetic bags, which are quite cheap and will keep their toilet articles tidy.

All patients should have as many baths as the staffing situation allows. Opportunities for good psychiatric nursing may be lost if baths have to be rushed because nurses have come to look on them as a tiresome chore, to be got through as quickly as possible.

One of the chief aims in the rehabilitation of regressed patients is to make them feel wanted and cared for. They are at a stage in their illness when, in some ways, their feelings are like those of children. Look back on the bath times of your own childhood—being allowed to have just five minutes more in the bath, the comfort of a crisp, clean bath towel, fresh underwear or pyjamas, tea or supper by the fire afterwards, the good physical pleasure of it all. Try to make bath time an occasion they look forward to.

It is often impossible to do all that we would like to do

and yet there are always a few nurses, in spite of staff shortages, who can find time for just that little extra which makes the difference between an impersonal routine and a therapeutic activity. Part of the skill of being a psychiatric nurse lies in seeing the value in simple things and being able to decide between those ward routines which really contribute to the patients' recovery and those which do not.

Entertainment. Evening entertainments will need to be held in the ward at first. Later, when patients have improved sufficiently to be transferred to another ward, they will be encouraged to go out in the evenings.

Community singing is generally popular. Let the patients choose the songs. It will help things along if you can get the words copied out and handed round so that everyone can join in. Dances are successful if you can coach a few patients beforehand, so that they and the nurses can start things off. Games evenings with whist or Bingo are enjoyed by most people.

Entertainments are opportunities to mix men and women by inviting a neighbouring ward to come over for the evening. It adds to the fun if a few simple prizes can be given. Many hospitals have funds for this purpose, or the League of Friends may be able to help. Ten cigarettes, a packet of chocolate, a pad of notepaper, a ballpoint pen, a comb or a tablet of soap can all be given to both men and women.

Talk about the evening in advance and get patients to help in the planning if possible. Allow plenty of time for washing and dressing before the visitors arrive and have a competition to see how many can make themselves smart enough to act as hosts and hostesses.

Personal relationships

In the field of personal relationships regressed patients need first to begin to feel like real individuals again, then to make contact with other people in the ward and in the hospital, and finally to get in touch with friends and relatives outside the hospital.

Every time a patient receives individual attention his self-respect is strengthened. The emphasis placed on physical care will contribute a great deal to this. Another way is to encourage him to have personal possessions whenever possible, particularly a personal issue of clothing and either his own clothes locker or a space for hanging clothes which is recognized as his. Birthdays are personal to everyone. This information is at hand in every ward. Mark the dates off on a calendar and have some little celebration every time a birthday comes along.

Making contact with other people may be difficult at first. A start can be made by encouraging patients to talk to one another. Ask a simple question, like 'Have you lived in Manchester all your life, Mr A?' and gradually draw the others in. Or use a game like 'I spy!' and break off for a chat about the object when someone has guessed it. Mixing men and women stimulates conversation. Sometimes people will talk more easily if you draw a few round the piano and start a sing-song. Patients who have been mute for years have been known to talk when pets were introduced into the ward, and budgerigars, goldfish or hamsters may help to bridge the gap. Aggressive patients are often noticeably gentle with pets.

Try to find out what relatives and friends the patient has and encourage him to write to them. Keeping in touch with relatives, or renewing the link if it has been broken, is of the utmost importance if the patient is to make his way back to the outside world and some time should be set aside in the ward programme each week specially for letter writing. See that part of the ward is quiet and that writing paper and pens are provided for those who do not have their own. Some patients may get stuck after 'Dear Mary', and need your help. One way is to suggest that the patient looks around him and describes the place in which he is sitting. For example

Dear Mary

I am sitting at the end of the ward in front of a big window. It is a beautiful day and I can see a bed of yellow roses in the garden.

I did enjoy your visit on Tuesday and hope you did too. Please come again when you can spare the time.

With love from

JACK

If the relative or friend has never visited him, or has not been for a long time, he might write the first paragraph as above and then say something like this

I have been thinking about you and wondering how you are. It seems a long time since I saw you and it would be lovely to hear from you. Please remember me to Tom and Peggy.

Yours ever

JACK

When visitors come to the ward go out of your way to make them as welcome as you can. Any questions about the patient's progress or the nature of his illness should be referred to charge nurse, but you can do a lot in other ways.

Go up to the visitor and introduce yourself as soon as he enters the ward. Don't leave him to wander round by himself looking for the patient.

When they are seated together leave them alone but keep a friendly eye on them. It can be an ordeal if you know nothing of mental illness and you are faced with someone who only says 'Yes' or 'No' and stares at the ground all the time. It often helps to break the ice if the visitor and the patient have something to do together, like having a cup of tea. The ward can usually supply this and if the patient is meeting his visitor in the social centre you can suggest that he takes enough money with him to buy tea at the canteen.

If you see they are not talking to each other stop in

passing and have a few words with them. 'Mr A, have you told Mrs B how you have been helping with the painting?' Or 'Miss G, have you shown your friend that lovely rug you are making?' Or suggest they might like to walk round the ward garden together. This will give them a topic to start on.

Tell the visitor a little of what goes on in the ward— the whist drive yesterday evening when patients from another ward came along, the trip to the hospital shop this afternoon. It is helpful for him to know that the patient does ordinary things like other people. Later, when the patient is better at letter writing, you can encourage him to put this kind of information in his letters.

A nurse who is off-hand and sits reading a newspaper all the time only confirms the visitor's fears that nothing can be done for the patient. A smart, alert nurse, with a pleasant manner, who shows that she is interested in the patient, creates an atmosphere of hopefulness in which improvement seems a possibility. Above all, be friendly. Make the visitor feel you are glad he has come and that you will welcome him next time.

When the visitor has left make a careful report of what you observed. Did he and the patient seem to get on well together? What did they talk about? Did they mention any other friends and relatives? What did the patient have to say after his visitor had left? This information can be helpful to sister, the doctor and the psychiatric social worker in their efforts to re-establish outside contacts for the patient.

If friends and relatives write to a patient who is not yet capable of writing back help him to read the letter and to understand who has written to him, then ask charge nurse if you may write back on his behalf. Give any messages you can from the patient and say how much the staff appreciate the writer's interest in him. Charge nurse will tell you what else to include in your letter.

This then is an outline of the methods you will use in

helping regressed patients. In time your group will be ready to move on to another ward, where they can learn to take more responsibility for themselves. You will be proud of the progress they have made and sorry to lose them, but don't hold them back. Without you these patients might never have started, but other people can carry on now. Wish them well and turn to the next group, who are waiting for you to help them over the first difficult steps.

INSTITUTIONALIZED PATIENTS

Seven out of every ten people admitted to a psychiatric hospital today will be discharged in a few months and many in six weeks or less thanks to modern methods of treatment, but this was not always possible in the past. In most hospitals there is a large group of patients who are not necessarily regressed or elderly but who have been in the hospital for many years, and are usually described as being institutionalized.

These people have made a life for themselves in the hospital, often in rather bizarre ways, and through no fault of their own are very resistant to change. Like regressed patients they have usually lost contact with any relatives they may have had, moreover they have no wish to meet them again. In fact they don't even want to leave the hospital, which has become an asylum to them in the true sense of the word, meaning a refuge or shelter. 'Madness' is their shield against the outside world and although most of them move freely about the hospital and the local town or village, they are unmistakably odd and are considered as such by the people they meet.

Most of the patients can, and do, wash, dress and feed themselves to acceptable social standards, yet they do not get on with normal people and in most cases appear to have lost the wish to do so. They seem to accept themselves as abnormal and often say, 'I'm mad, dear. I know

I'm mad', as though this is an affliction they are saddled with, which effectively cuts them off from those who are 'not mad', as indeed it does.

The majority of them are neither demented nor old, being very often in their 40's or 50's. Few of them see a doctor more than twice a year and almost all have been written off as psychiatrically of no interest, so whatever is done to help them to a fuller, richer and more normal life will have to be done by nurses—with no extra money or staff to help them. The most we can hope for is better drugs but many of these patients have little medication anyway.

So what can we do to help them? Physically they are able to care for themselves, although the nurses' continued interest is necessary to help them modify some of their more unusual forms of dress and behaviour and to make the best of their appearance. Their main needs lie in the fields of work, leisure and personal relationships.

Work

Some patients will start by working in one of the hospital departments. They might be laundry maids, porters, needlewomen, kitchen hands, gardeners, clerks, typists, cleaners, or messengers. A dressmaker who could take up her work again when she leaves hospital might be helped by working in the sewing room. Clerks and typists can polish up their skills by working in the various offices.

Others, who perhaps have no particular training, may be helped by attending the industrial unit. This is a department which does simple assembly work for local factories, such as putting together display boxes, fancy goods, souvenirs, pens, drawing kits, pencil boxes, cardboard packing boxes, and toys of all kinds. Nurses and occupational therapists work with the patients in this department.

By working in hospital departments or in the industrial

unit patients gradually get used to the conditions they will meet when they finally leave hospital.

They have to get to the place where they work at the right time. Their work must be up to standard or it is not accepted and in industrial therapy they must work at the same pace as the next man or they will put the whole line out. Men and women get used to working side by side after perhaps having been in separate wards for a long time. They can see that they are doing real work, which needs to be done, and this proves to them that they are of value to the community.

Their pay packets at the end of the week show them that their value is recognized. Pay increases according to the amount of effort they put into their work. This encourages them to do better, and the fact that they are truly earning the money helps them to regain a feeling of independence and self-respect.

When you are with patients in the industrial unit you must first learn how to do the work yourself and make certain you understand what the factory wants. Once you are thoroughly familiar with the task to be done you can join with the rest of the team to help the patients.

You will find that the work can be broken up into a number of simple steps. For instance, in assembling a paper carrier bag you could make twelve to fifteen different movements. This is useful because it means the team can organize the work to suit the patients' abilities. Some may only be able to make one movement, such as folding the paper in half, or brushing one strip with glue, or pressing the glued strip down. In that case you will have a group of patients of about the same ability, each contributing one movement as the carrier bags move round the table. Others may be able to do six or seven of the movements. For example, one will do all the folding, another apply all the glue and a third will finish it off. These people can complete the bags by working in groups of three. Those who are capable of making the whole bag unaided are ready to move on to something a little more complicated.

As you help the patients you should watch them carefully. Are they able to concentrate on the job? Can they keep up an even pace? Someone who gets anxious about keeping up may need an easier task, while the patient who gets irritable because the others keep him waiting may be able to move to a group where he has more to do. How well does the excitable patient get on with his neighbours, is he a cheerful influence or a constant annoyance, preventing them from doing their best? The patient who hears voices—does he carry on with his work unconcerned or does he have to stop every few minutes to listen? Is the withdrawn patient able to keep his mind on what he is doing or does he keep wandering off into his private world? Perhaps it will help if you speak to him every few minutes or so. Notice if you can lengthen the time as the days go by and his concentration improves.

The reason for finding patients work to do, whether in a hospital department or in the industrial unit, is that they should finally be able to leave the hospital entirely and support themselves in the community. So the ward team meets frequently to assess their progress and plan the next steps in their rehabilitation.

These meetings are called case conferences and the people that might be present include nurses, occupational therapists, the patient's doctor, the social worker. A nursing officer and one of the tutors may also be able to take part. Everyone contributes what he knows about the patient's special problems, his aptitudes and what progress he has made so far. Your own observations will be valuable, and when you know a case conference is to be held you should re-read your Nurses' Notes on the patient and try to recall anything else which may help the team in its discussion.

If a patient is thought to be ready to try to find work

outside the hospital the disablement resettlement officer
may be asked to give his advice. He is a member of the
staff of the local labour exchange. He is specially appointed by the Department of Employment and Productivity
to help people who are recovering from illness, either mental or physical, and who, because of their illness, are disabled temporarily or permanently. He is in close touch
with all the employers in the district and knows what work
is available. The ward team will discuss the patient with
him and if he knows of a suitable vacancy he will help the
patient to apply for the job.

Patients who work outside the hospital may continue
to live in the ward for a while. Each morning after breakfast they go off to work, returning to the ward in the
evening. In this way they still have the support of the
ward team while getting used to life outside. They get the
full union rates of pay and pay a fixed sum to the hospital
for their board and lodging.

Leisure

Institutionalized patients often become so accustomed
to having entertainments organized for them that they
lose the initiative to make arrangements for themselves.

They need to be helped in every way possible to regain
this initiative.

A ward party once a week is an opportunity to invite
patients from another ward and to mix men and women,
but all the organization should be done by the patients.
Your task will be to start them thinking and to show them
how they can arrange it for themselves.

With charge nurse's approval they should find out
whether the evening they have chosen is convenient for
the other ward and issue their own invitations. They
should plan the programme. If games are part of the plan
see that they themselves count the packs of cards, check
the draughts and get out the table-tennis set. If there is to
be dancing let them select the records, decide who will put

them on and choose their own master of ceremonies. Later, when the visitors have gone, they should help in tidying the ward and putting everything away before they go to bed.

Although a weekly social event in the ward may be helpful the patients need to go outside the hospital as much as possible during the rest of their free time.

Encourage them to go to the cinema in the evenings, to the public library, to exhibitions or to the theatre, and help them make the arrangements themselves. For instance if a patient wants to know what is on at the cinema, don't say 'Oh, I'll find out for you', but 'Now I wonder how we can find out?' If he has no idea at all suggest the local paper, but let him, and the other patients, find out for themselves. Perhaps they could telephone the cinema. Show them where the telephone directories are kept, but let them look up the number and make the call themselves. If they are going to the theatre let them ring up and make inquiries about booking seats. Be at hand all the time in case they meet a difficulty, but give them only just enough help to take the next step on their own.

You will find, of course, that this takes up far more of your time than doing it for them, and when you are busy you will often be tempted to give patients information or to do things for them simply because it is quicker that way. Try not to do this. Good nursing means making it possible for the patient to help himself. There is an art in guiding him without embarrassing him. Don't treat him like a child and stand over him as it were. Join in doing things with him all the time but contrive that he should appear to take the lead. When you become accustomed to this you will be amply rewarded by the pleasure that returning self-confidence can bring to the patient.

Encourage patients to use the hospital's social centre. Here they can meet people from other wards, talk, listen to music, play games, entertain their visitors in the café, buy a paper, get a few items from the shop. In other words they can begin to feel something of what it is like to be in the general community again.

At weekends many patients will go on leave or out for the day with relatives and friends. Those who are unable to do so can go out in small groups with a nurse, shopping in the town, going on a picnic or a country walk, or perhaps going off for the day to some place of interest.

Sometimes patients from several wards are collected together to be taken out in a coach for a day at the sea, or for a country drive. Although this is much better than letting them remain idle in the wards it is even more helpful if they can go in small groups of four or five with a nurse.

The small group is so much more personal. When twenty or thirty patients are taken out at a time the organization is done by the hospital and they are transported from door to door. The outing is pleasant, but their contribution is largely a passive one. A small group can go by bus and train. The patients, with your help, can look up the times of trains, find out where changes have to be made, decide what time the return journey will have to begin, get their own tickets, find their own seats, remember the way back from the beach to the railway station. All this is just as enjoyable and far more therapeutic because these are the ordinary activities which people outside hospital take for granted but which cause institutionalized patients so much anxiety when they are discharged.

Other activities at the weekend can include buying food and cooking. A small group of patients left in the ward when others are on leave could make jam tarts for Sunday tea. Eggs and bacon, bought by themselves and cooked over the ward gas ring, may not be as elaborate as the roast pork with all its trimmings from the main kitchen, but again it will be a chance to re-learn something which is part of the business of everyday life and this is what institutionalized patients need.

Knowledge of current affairs is important. Someone who gets a job in the district will be thought a bit odd by his workmates if he isn't aware of the latest political scandal or the state of the league tables, not to mention the more serious news.

Encourage patients to listen regularly to the news bulletins and discussion programmes on radio and television. Listen with them and talk about what is happening. Read the newspapers with them and get them discussing the day's headlines. Find a dictionary and an atlas to keep in the ward and make a game of 'Let's look that one up!' Look at the situations vacant column in the local paper and talk about different jobs and how people apply for them.

Personal relationships

Not only do institutionalized patients need to recall old skills, they must also learn how to get on with other people again. This is another part of life which has become difficult for them.

Contact with relatives and friends is important. If you make visitors feel welcome in the ward they are more likely to come regularly. This gives an opportunity for the patient and his relatives to get used to one another again. It may have been a long while since they saw each other and they need time to get acquainted.

Another way of bringing them together is to invite relatives and friends to a social evening in the ward. This also allows the staff to observe how they react to each other. Do they seem at ease, do they talk together amicably or are there arguments? Does the visitor seem to be irritated, or anxious, or frightened by what the patient says and does? Is the patient relaxed after the visit or does he seem tense or depressed? Keep your eyes and ears open and report what you notice. All this information will help in deciding what is best for the patient.

Some patients will have no visitors and here the League of Friends may be able to help. Often a member is willing to take two or three patients out for a meal, or to his home for an afternoon.

Here again you can help by making the member feel that the staff appreciate his offer. When he meets the patient for the first time sit and talk with them both for a little while. This will make it easier for them to get to know each other. If the patient has any strange mannerisms or ideas which might worry the visitor he will learn what to do by seeing how you behave towards the patient.

These patients can only be as independent as we allow them to be, and the level of independence allowed by most hospitals is far too low. Institutionalized patients are the victims of the hospital's state of institutionalization, rather than the chronic nature of their own illness, and too many of them spend their lives in a state of such suffocating boredom that it would drive people less brainwashed by the system either to despair or to violent protest.

What they need more than anything else is to be cared about and treated as if they were human beings and to be encouraged to do things for themselves.

Try to make at least one individual, personal contact with each patient, every day—remembering that it's his birthday, telling him a small personal joke or bit of information, getting him to help you in some individual activity. 'I wish you'd give me a hand to sort these books.' Anything that is personal between you, as a nurse and this particular patient. It is time we realized how desperate is the need and longing of chronic patients to be treated differently, to be made to feel special, to be given individual notice and attention. One of the sad things about such patients is the ease with which they can come and go unseen. It is so easy to ignore them, or if we don't ignore them, to treat them as if they were cardboard cutouts to be moved about at our convenience, rather than flesh and blood people.

These are patients who need to be addressed by their own name, clothed in their own clothing, given their own lockers, involved in a personal way with each other and with the staff. They need opportunities to learn some simple activity, choose a hobby and make friends. The men need their pint of bitter and a seat in the sun. The women need attractive clothes and an occasional outing, just like men and women outside. This will do more for them than any drug, and it is in your power to give it to them, if you will make the effort.

Ward meetings are as important for long-stay patients as they are for patients who are only in the hospital for a short time.

Discussion with patients can show the ward team what progress is being made and what problems remain to be solved. It also gives patients an opportunity to express themselves. As they talk, and listen to others talking, they may be able to sort out some of their difficulties. The feeling of sharing gives patients and staff a sense of belonging to a community and working together towards the patients' discharge. As most of the patients will be at work during the day it may not be convenient to hold ward meetings in the morning but it is usually quite possible to fit them in during the evenings.

As always, ward meetings need to be followed by staff meetings. Active rehabilitation calls for constant adjustment by the staff to the patients' needs. Gradually the ward team has to withdraw its support so that the patient can stand on his own feet, but just how to do this, and to what extent for each patient, needs much thought. Sometimes ward routine is upset and this can be annoying. Patients, feeling their independence, may break some of the ward rules and the nurses may not be sure what to do about it. When progress seems to be slow staff may feel discouraged and lose their enthusiasm.

Frank discussion of these and similar problems helps the members of the ward staff to come to an understanding with each other and to plan a common policy so that everyone can work together as a real team for the good of the patients.

12

Patients with organic disorders

You will find that some patients in psychiatric hospitals are suffering from a disease or disorder of the brain as well as being mentally ill. They have been admitted for treatment of the mental illness, but in most cases this illness has developed from the physical and psychological stresses of the organic disorder and the patient has the double burden of his mental illness and his physical condition. Examples of such diseases or disorders of the brain are epilepsy, Parkinsonism, general paresis and Huntington's chorea. Perhaps the ones you will meet most often are the patients with epilepsy.

EPILEPSY

Our brains are made up of myriads of cells. Each cell gives off a tiny electric current. This is normal and goes on all through our lives. In some people the cells suddenly give off a much greater electric current and the person may have an epileptic fit.

We do not know exactly why the brain cells do this. Some people have fits as children and continue to do so all their lives. Often no cause can be found. Others start having fits after developing a tumour in the brain or after some injury to the brain. Sometimes old people suffering from arteriosclerosis will start having fits.

We do not yet know the cure for epilepsy, but it can

be controlled by drugs and sometimes an operation to remove part of the temporal lobe, which lies underneath that section of the skull which is just above the ear, is successful in stopping fits. Although their fits can be controlled by drugs, many epileptic people cannot be persuaded to take their tablets regularly while they are at home. Because they haven't had a fit for some time they think that they are cured and stop taking them. Unfortunately this is not so, and they will certainly begin to have fits again if they do this. However, with regular medication they can lead practically normal lives, and you are unlikely to see many patients having fits in hospital.

PARKINSONISM

Another large group are those suffering from Parkinsonism. This illness is caused by an infection of the cells at the base of the brain, and there is no known cure for it.

The patient is unable to control his limbs properly. His arms and legs gradually become rigid and sometimes a fine tremor develops in his hands, so that he has difficulty in holding anything and is always dropping things. He has a shuffling kind of walk, often teetering along on tiptoe and looking as if he is going to fall forward on his face at any moment. His face itself lacks expression and can become almost like a mask, with saliva dribbling from his lips. In addition his eyes may turn in one direction, usually upwards, and remain so for periods varying from a few seconds to an hour or more. This movement of the eyes is called an oculogyric crisis. These symptoms gradually increase over the years, until the patient is helpless and bedridden.

A similar group of symptoms can arise in patients who are being given tranquillizing drugs, such as chlorpromazine, but these symptoms disappear when the patient is taken off the drug. There is a growing number of patients like this in psychiatric hospitals where tranquillizing drugs are widely used and among the general public Parkinsonism due to brain infection also seems to be on the increase.

GENERAL PARESIS

A smaller group are those patients suffering from general paresis.

General paresis is caused by syphilis affecting the cells of the brain. The patient may be irritable, confused, depressed, unable to concentrate for any length of time, dirty in his habits and slovenly in appearance. He may imagine that he is a person of great importance or that he owns a great deal of money and can buy anything he wants. These ideas are called delusions of grandeur. He often has an unsteady, staggering kind of walk, finds it difficult to speak or write clearly, and in the later stages of the illness he may be incontinent and bedridden.

Again there is no cure for this disease, but large doses of penicillin may stop it becoming worse.

You are unlikely to see many patients with general paresis nowadays because syphilis is so easily cured in its early stages that there is little danger of the infection reaching the brain, but before the discovery of penicillin there were many of these people in mental hospitals and the illness was known as general paralysis of the insane. This was shortened to the initials G.P.I. and you may perhaps hear members of the staff referring to a patient as suffering from 'G.P.I.'

General paresis is of special interest to psychiatric nurses because it was one of the first mental illnesses for which an effective treatment was discovered. Ask any of the older members of the staff about malarial therapy for G.P.I. You will be fascinated at what they have to tell you.

HUNTINGTON'S CHOREA

Huntington's chorea is a rare disease, but you will probably meet one or two patients suffering from this tragic illness. Again it is caused by a disorder of the brain cells. The patient develops abrupt, jerking and stretching movements of his arms which are beyond his control and that go on all the time he is awake. Later there is writhing of the face and trunk and repeated sniffing and snorting. As the disease progresses still further his speech is affected and may become incomprehensible, until finally he is completely helpless.

Huntington's chorea is inherited. If one of the parents has the disease then fifty per cent of their children are sure to develop it. If you think about this for a moment you will realize what an appalling burden these people carry.

Suppose a man knows that the disease is in his family. There is a fifty-fifty chance he will get it himself. His mother or father has it, and he watches them become increasingly grotesque and helpless as the years go by, knowing that this is what will probably happen to him too. Perhaps he marries. Dare he have children? If he does he knows that they also have a fifty-fifty chance of getting the disease. So he watches every tiny symptom, every ache and pain, in himself and in the children, dreading that it may mean the onset of the disease.

If he develops Huntington's chorea himself, he knows his children will have to watch him die slowly over the years, thinking all the time that this is how they will most likely end up themselves. No wonder these people become severely depressed and sometimes feel like committing suicide.

Epileptic people, provided that they take their drugs regularly, are hardly handicapped at all by their condition, and if those you meet in hospital seem to be suspicious, irritable, bad-tempered, or lazy, these characteristics are more likely to be symptoms of the mental illness for which they have been admitted, than the result of their epilepsy. Fortunately the general public has a more enlightened attitude towards epilepsy than was the case some years ago and although there is still a certain amount of prejudice against them, most people feel sympathetic towards epileptics and try to help them.

Patients suffering from general paresis, Parkinsonism and Huntington's chorea will all show an increasing loss of intellectual ability, due to the deterioration of their brain cells. They gradually become slow and muddled in their thinking. They forget where they are and what day it is. Sometimes they misunderstand what is going on around them. For example, they may think the doctors and nurses are members of their family. Their memory begins to fail, especially for recent events, although they may still be able to recall accurately what happened twenty or thirty years ago. This gradual decline is called dementia and patients with epilepsy may also become demented if their fits are not controlled. As you would expect, these patients often become depressed, particularly those suffering from Parkinsonism and Huntington's chorea. Patients with Parkinsonism may show signs of acute anxiety as well at times.

People who have a disability which cannot be cured need to come to terms with their difficulties if they are to live their lives as fully as possible. But it is one thing to adjust yourself to the loss of a leg or an arm, or even to the loss of sight or hearing, and quite another to realize that you will gradually lose all control of your body and your mind and that you will end up as a burden to yourself and all around you.

As their disease progresses it becomes impossible for the patients we have been considering to continue working; even keeping a few friends and leading something approaching a normal life may soon be beyond them. Trying to help these people is not so much a test of our nursing skill as of our imagination and compassion, as human beings.

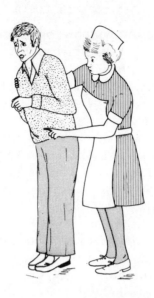

It means making time to wait while they get out the slow muddled words they are trying to say. It means helping them to join in what is going on whenever possible, but always shielding them from what is beyond their strength, either mentally or physically and above all having the sensitivity to save them from embarrassment. It means the ready smile and greeting each time you go by, even if they never respond; the friendly hand on his shoulder, or your arm slipped through hers for a moment. Inside the shuffling, jerking body and behind the drooling face and dull eyes, is a relatively normal person who longs more than anything else for human contact and ordinary human kindness. When you feel disgusted and repelled by what you see, try to remember that this is only the cage. Trapped inside is someone just like you and me.

DIAGNOSTIC TESTS

One diagnostic test which is often used by the doctor in connection with organic disorders is the EEG, or electroencephalogram.

This is a record on a sheet of paper of the minute electric currents coming from the brain cells. It looks something like a temperature chart and gives the doctor useful information about whether the patient has a tendency to epileptic fits. He can also tell what type of epilepsy the patient is suffering from. Most EEGs are painless but a few, while not being actually painful, are acutely unpleasant.

When a patient is to have an EEG try to find out what he thinks it is and how he feels about it. If he is fearful, or misinformed, do your best to reassure him. Tell him that everyone's brain gives out small electric impulses. This is perfectly normal and goes on all the time. When a doctor wants to magnify a patient's heartbeat he listens to it through a stethoscope. When he wants to magnify the impulses from a patient's brain he uses the electro-encephalogram machine. Several small electrodes are fixed to the patient's head and by this means the impulses are recorded in the form of a graph on a piece of paper. Fixing the electrodes does not hurt at all. The patient is not having electricity passed through his brain. The doctor cannot read his thoughts. In fact, nothing is being done to the patient other than making a record of the impulses which are coming from his brain all the time.

Lumbar puncture

Another test you may sometimes hear mentioned is the lumbar puncture.

The brain and spinal cord are constantly bathed in fluid. A sample of this fluid can be obtained by inserting a special lumbar puncture needle in the lower part of the patient's back between the bones of the spine.

If the patient has a disease of the brain, or of the spinal cord, certain changes take place in this fluid which can be ascertained by examining a sample.

As with an EEG, this test is not painful. The patient usually lies on his left side, the doctor gives him a local anaesthetic in the small of his back, and then takes the sample. The patient feels nothing but the small prick of the local anaesthetic.

Occasionally patients have a headache after this test, but in most cases it can be prevented by seeing that they lie down somewhere quiet after the test is over and stay there for two or three hours.

13

Psychopathic personality, drug and alcohol dependence and sexual disorders

You will meet some patients in the hospital who are not suffering from any known mental disorder but their behaviour is of a kind that the majority of people are unable to tolerate and it is thought that medical treatment may help them.

Some of these patients realize that they need help and come into hospital of their own accord. Others do not wish to change their way of life, but they have been forced to enter hospital either because they have come into conflict with the law or because they are a danger to themselves or others.

PSYCHOPATHIC PATIENTS

A psychopathic patient seems to be unable to control his desires. Whatever he wants he will try to get, regardless of other people and without concern for the long-term effect on himself. He will steal, lie and take advantage of others, without apparently feeling any guilt, and with little thought of the consequences.

Although he may cause himself trouble by his behaviour he seems unable to learn from his mistakes and punishment appears to have no effect on him.

His relationships with other people are shallow and he breaks a relationship as soon as he can no longer get what he wants from the other person.

When they cannot have what they want some psychopathic patients become violently angry. These patients are described as aggressive psychopaths. Others seem to be quite incapable of running their lives without the constant help of everyone around them and are known as inadequate psychopaths.

Doctors are not yet certain about what causes psychopathic behaviour and they are not entirely decided on how to treat it. Some think the answer lies in firm discipline, with rewards for acceptable behaviour and penalties when rules are broken. Others feel that these patients should be treated in a more permissive way, but made to face up to the consequences of their behaviour and to deal with it. At the same time they should be helped, through discussion with the staff and other patients, to understand why they behave as they do.

You may find doctors treating psychopathic patients in various ways, but one principle remains constant throughout—whatever plan is adopted it is essential that the ward staff should act together as a team.

When you first meet a psychopathic patient he may appear quite charming. He is interested in you as a person, wants to know what your opinion is on this and that, and offers to help with the ward work. He obviously admires your ability as a nurse and understands how other people do not always appreciate your worth. Soon he is using your Christian name and asking little favours of you. He is so pleasant and helpful that it is hard to refuse. In any case you feel that you understand his needs perhaps better than anyone else in the ward and that anything you can do to strengthen the nurse-patient relationship between you will be for his good. So you save his breakfast for him when he doesn't feel like getting up with the others. You make excuses for him when he is late returning from leave. You clear up the mess round his locker because he will be so hurt if you don't.

When he suddenly stops coming to you and you hear he has been making disparaging remarks about you to another nurse you feel desperately let down.

In other words, psychopathic patients are past-masters at using other people to their own advantage.

Like all patients the psychopathic patient needs you to be interested in him. He needs your concern and your attention. He needs you to accept him without judgement and to be prepared to like him. But it is one thing to understand how a patient feels and quite another to feel whatever the patient wants you to feel.

If his experience in the past has convinced him that everyone can be bribed, flattered, or bullied into doing what he wants, it will not help him at all to come into hospital and find that these tactics work with the hospital staff too.

Once a patient can control your reaction to him you can no longer help him. On the other hand if you can like the person behind the difficult behaviour and go on quietly wishing him well even when his hostility is deliberately aimed at you, then you may be able to do a lot for him. This is true of all patients, but it is nowhere more obvious than in the care of psychopathic patients.

Resist the temptation to go it alone with a psycho-pathic patient. You may be right in thinking you understand him better than anyone else, but don't keep it to yourself. Tell the rest of the ward team at the staff meetings and be guided by what they decide should be done.

Often some line of action which you feel will help the patient may seem to conflict with your responsibilities towards the other patients, and it is only by discussion with the rest of the team that you and everyone else can arrive at what is the best thing to do.

Psychopathic patients are specialists at stirring up rivalry, tension, suspicion and misunderstanding between other people. This is how they have made their way through life so far. If we are to help them alter their behaviour then we must be proof against their methods ourselves, and we can only do this by having the courage to tell each other when we feel angry or jealous or hurt, and being willing to talk it over together, as a team.

If we can support each other in this way whatever plan of treatment we decide upon has a far better chance of success.

DRUG AND ALCOHOL DEPENDENCE

The two most common forms of dependence found in psychiatric hospitals are dependence on drugs and dependence on alcohol.

Patients dependent on drugs

A person may take to drugs in the first place because he is depressed or anxious and finds they give him a lift. He may try it out of curiosity, or because he wants to keep in with the rest of his group, or because he can't sleep. As time goes by he finds that when he stops taking the drug he feels even worse than he did before. So he goes on.

Gradually he has to take larger and larger doses to get the same effect. This is called *tolerance*. Buying the drug begins to be expensive, but by this time he can't do without it. He has developed an *intense craving* for it. Nothing else matters except the next dose, and he will do anything to get it. He lies and steals to get the money, loses his job and begins to lead a kind of twilight existence. He doesn't bother to eat, wash or change his clothes. His health deteriorates. By this time he cannot stop taking the drug and he doesn't want to. It is beyond his control and he has become an addict.

When people who are addicted to drugs suddenly stop taking them they may suffer from *withdrawal symptoms*, particularly if they have been taking morphine or heroin. These include confusion, fits, muscular spasms, abdominal cramp, sweating, restlessness, sleeplessness and depression. In a person whose physical health is already poor they can be dangerously exhausting.

The term 'addiction' should only be used when these three aspects, namely tolerance, intense craving for the drug, and withdrawal symptoms, are present.

Treatment for these patients is aimed at preventing them from taking the drug, trying to show them a more constructive way of dealing with their problems, and building up their physical health.

The doctor may order the drug to be stopped altogether, or he may order it to be withdrawn gradually over a period of a week or more to reduce the severity of the withdrawal symptoms. Sometimes he may wean the patient off the drug by substituting a less harmful one, or by giving him modified insulin therapy (see Chapter Seventeen).

When such a patient is admitted always assume that he has brought drugs in with him, no matter what he says to the contrary.

He will probably be very much in need of a bath so while your colleague helps him in the bathroom take all his clothes, and anything else he has brought in, and search until you find them. He will not, of course, try to hide them in his pockets where you would be sure to find them, and you will have to make a thorough search of hems, linings, turnups, seams, belts, and so on, until you are certain you have missed nothing.

During the withdrawal period he will be nursed in bed and will need all the basic nursing care you would give to a seriously ill patient. Withdrawal symptoms can be severe and you may think that the patient's craving is so strong that it is inhuman to deny him a small amount of the drug. This is false kindness and would only prolong his distress. Support him in every way you can, by being with him and by assuring him that the symptoms will pass.

When he is able to get up again he will need plenty of fresh air and exercise, a nourishing diet and a full programme of occupation.

If he is allowed visitors remember that they too may have drugs, however strongly they deny it, and they will probably try to get some in for him. Use all your skill to prevent the patient receiving a fresh supply. Once he starts taking drugs again all the good will be undone and the craving will return. His only hope lies in complete abstinence and an intensive plan for rehabilitation.

Patients dependent on alcohol

Most of us have felt all the better for a drink on occasions. Alcohol can help a shy person to feel confident, it can lift depression and relieve tension. Many people drink heavily and enjoy it.

Some people drink not for enjoyment but because they cannot face life without alcohol. This kind of drinker finds that as time goes by he needs more and more to get the same relief. He tries to hide his drinking from others but his health begins to break down. He lies and blusters, but his wife is not deceived. There are bitter quarrels, the children are frightened. He loses his job and the family breaks up. He knows what he is doing to the people he loves, but he can't stop because he is addicted and he drinks even more to blot out his guilt and depression until he makes himself a mental and physical wreck.

Sometimes alcoholics can be persuaded to seek help before they reach this stage, but many are not ready to do so until they have ruined their own lives and brought misery to their families.

When the patient comes into hospital he is allowed no alcohol at all and this sudden withdrawal may cause symptoms similar to those following the withdrawal of drugs. Again we have the picture of tolerance, intense craving, and withdrawal symptoms.

Occasionally a patient may suffer from delirium tremens (DTs). This is a dreadful experience for him. He is restless, confused and feverish, and has horrifying hallucinations, frequently of animals. We may joke about seeing pink elephants, but the reality is a nightmare. Like the patient who is dependent on drugs he needs intensive nursing care during this stage. See that he has as little stimulation as possible because he is so frightened. Keep your voice quiet, but speak clearly. Avoid talking to other people in tones he cannot hear as it will only add to his fear. Because he is so terrified it may help him if you leave the light on all the time.

Very often the alcohol has poisoned his nervous system so that he does not feel heat or cold as acutely as healthy people do. Unless you are specially told to do so by charge nurse it is best not to give him a hot-water bottle because it is so easy to burn him.

The alcohol also destroys vitamins in his body. His doctor will want him to have a light diet, with extra vitamins either by mouth or by injection, and plenty of fluids. He may also order drugs which will calm him.

There are two drugs which are sometimes used to help these patients to overcome their addiction.

Apomorphine is a drug which induces nausea and vomiting. The patient is given an injection of apomorphine and at the same time he is allowed a drink of alcohol. No sooner has he taken the drink than he is violently sick. This treatment is repeated every two hours for three days. During this time the patient is given injections of vitamin B, but nothing to eat or drink except alcohol, and each time he takes alcohol he vomits.

This is called aversion therapy, because the doctor hopes to build up an aversion to alcohol by forcing the patient to associate drink with nausea, vomiting and extreme discomfort.

The patient rapidly becomes exhausted. There is a danger that he will suffer heart failure, or that repeated vomiting will cause bleeding from his stomach (haematemesis). His temperature, pulse, respiration and blood pressure are recorded every two hours, and his urine tested twice a day for sugar and acetone. The doctor is always within immediate call and the nurse must let him know at once if the patient shows signs of shock—falling blood pressure, weak, rapid pulse, restlessness, pallor, and cold, clammy skin.

If all goes well the patient starts to take ordinary food at the end of the third day and the injections of apomorphine are gradually reduced over the next two days.

The second drug is *Antabuse*. If the patient takes Antabuse and then has a drink he feels hot, his heart races, he is breathless and he has a pounding headache. If he persists in taking more alcohol he vomits and may collapse, but the symptoms following the first drink are usually enough to prevent him taking another.

He can be up and about, leading an ordinary life and eating a normal diet while having the treatment, but he must take the drug regularly for at least a year, or until he has lost all desire for alcohol.

Another source of help for alcoholics is a society called *Alcoholics Anonymous* (AA).

This is a voluntary association of people who have already recovered from addiction to alcohol, or are in the process of recovering. In the fellowship of AA members do their utmost to support each other in every possible way to resist the temptation to take 'just a little one'. Alcoholism is a disease and the alcoholic must never touch drink again if he is to recover. It is the first drink which does the damage every time. Members are on call to each other at any time of the day or night, and since they have been through similar experiences they find a sense of community and support through their membership which they cannot get outside. In addition there is a strong religious element in the society which many alcoholics find helpful.

Patients who suffer from any form of dependence present a difficult problem for the ward team. The only real hope of recovery lies in the patient's wish to get better. Unfortunately, by the very fact that he has become dependent, he not only cannot give up the drug or the drink, but he doesn't really want to. What he would like is to be freed of his guilt and left in peace with an unlimited source of supply.

Reproaches and good advice are of no use whatever. Family and friends have tried to help him in this way, perhaps for years. Often he is himself a harsher judge of his actions than anyone else and his own guilt overwhelms him.

What he needs is a relationship that remains constant in spite of all setbacks. The nurse can make such a relationship with him, but only if she realizes that he is suffering from an illness.

It is not a question of will power, or of pulling himself together, or of having a little decency, or sparing a thought for his wife and family, and so on. You might as well blame someone with tonsillitis for having an infected throat as blame an addict for breaking good resolutions. He will tell you one thing and do another. Full of optimism and plans for the future one day he will be morose and hostile or full of self-pity and excuses the next. Take care not to let yourself be cast up and down in sympathy. Try to realize that these are the symptoms of an illness.

If you and the patient can take a good look at these symptoms together, and if you can remain interested in him and understanding, in spite of the setbacks, you will be playing an important part in the team effort which is needed to bring him back to health.

SEXUAL DISORDERS

Sexual disorder is a condition in which a person is unable to achieve sexual satisfaction through normal intercourse, either because of impotence or frigidity, or because his sexual needs and drives are not directed towards normal sexual intercourse.

A man or woman may attempt normal intercourse and have difficulty in carrying it through to a climax. The man is either unable to sustain an erection or he ejaculates too soon. This is called impotence. The woman is unable to achieve a climax. This is called frigidity.

Impotence and frigidity are often caused by anxiety, depression, or ignorance, but in some cases they may be the result of psychological difficulties in early childhood.

Sexual deviation

A man or a woman may find sexual satisfaction from practices which do not end in normal intercourse. This is called sexual deviation. Sexual deviation may be caused by psychological problems arising from experiences in childhood. It can also occur as a result of diseases affecting the nervous system or the endocrine balance of the body.

There are many deviations and the same person may practice more than one of them. Among the more common are the following.

Homosexuality is attraction towards a person of the same sex. It is normal during adolescence, but abnormal if it continues into adult life.

Most people think of a male homosexual as looking effeminate, with a mincing walk and a high-pitched voice, but this is rare. Most male homosexuals are masculine in appearance. Similarly the mannish woman with short hair, who wears a tweed suit with collar and tie, is far outnumbered by the female homosexual who, to all appearances, is just like other women.

A male homosexual may practise intercourse by inserting his penis into his partner's anus, but the most common practice among male or female homosexuals is mutual masturbation.

Some homosexuals are promiscuous. Many form temporary liaisons with other homosexuals. A few may form stable partnerships which last for a number of years and many are able to lead reasonably well-adjusted lives. It is only the minority who have to come into hospital.

Many people are attracted to both men and women, that is to say they are both homosexual and heterosexual, but usually one attraction is stronger than the other.

Paedophilia is the desire to make sexual advances to children. The paedophiliac is nearly always a man, although very occasionally women have been known to suffer from this deviation. The general public gets the impression that the rape of little girls is common because every case receives the full attention of the press, but in fact intercourse is rare. The man usually masturbates the child, or persuades the child to masturbate him.

Exhibitionism is almost entirely confined to men. The man has a desire to show his penis to women or little girls and obtains satisfaction from their reaction of shock or excitement. Contrary to popular belief he rarely makes any attempt to touch the woman.

Voyeurism is the desire to watch people of the opposite sex in the nude, or while having intercourse. It is more common in men than in women and Peeping Toms probably suffer from this deviation.

Fetishism is a condition in which the person gets sexual satisfaction from certain objects. It is chiefly confined to men, and common objects used are women's underclothing, furs or shoes.

Sadism is the desire to inflict pain and *masochism* is the desire to submit to pain. Sadists and masochists get sexual satisfaction through inflicting or submitting to pain. Both characteristics may occur together in the same person.

Transvestism is the experience of sexual satisfaction from the wearing of clothes of the opposite sex.

In a normal sexual relationship both the man and the woman get satisfaction from seeing one another unclothed. Different parts of the body rouse sexual desire, there is a wish to dominate the partner or to surrender and be dominated. All these aspects of sexual behaviour are normal if they lead to intercourse. They only become abnormal when they are an end in themselves and the people concerned have no wish for normal intercourse.

The word deviation means a turning aside. The sexual deviant has turned aside from the broad highway of normal sex by taking one small part of sexual behaviour and trying to get all his satisfaction from that only. He is walking down a blind alley.

Sexual disorder is not a sin—it is a great misfortune. The deviant does not deliberately set out to act in a perverse manner because he is wicked, or enjoys wickedness. Many people who are able to achieve full satisfaction through normal sexual intercourse do not fully appreciate the power of the sexual drive in human nature.

Those who do not achieve normal intercourse, either by reason of impotence or frigidity, or because they are sexual deviants, are often extremely lonely people. The intensity of their sexual needs may drive them into a form of behaviour which they themselves often deplore, but which they are unable to give up.

One of the difficulties in trying to help deviants is that although they may be frustrated and unhappy they often have no true desire to change because their deviation is their only means of satisfaction.

People who are suffering from sexual disorder as a result of ignorance or anxiety can often be helped by attending an outpatient clinic where they can talk freely to the doctor and receive advice. They will probably not need to come into hospital.

If the disorder is the result of deep-seated problems they may still be helped by frequent interviews with the doctor as outpatients, but the process is usually slow and treatment must continue over a long period to be successful. Occasionally stilboestrol, which is one of the female sex hormones, is given to men to reduce their sexual drive. This may be helpful, for instance, to a man suffering from paedophilia.

Those who come into hospital usually do so because they are too depressed or too anxious, as a result of their disorder, to be able to carry on their lives outside. Some doctors use aversion therapy for deviations, so that the patient comes to associate extreme physical discomfort with his sexual practices, but the effect may not last for any length of time. For most patients who come into hospital treatment is aimed at relieving their depression and anxiety and helping them to adjust to their disability.

Probably the kind of deviation you will meet most frequently in hospital is homosexuality.

A male homosexual will look on a male nurse or a male doctor as a possible sexual partner, but he will think of a female nurse either as his sister or as his mother. He will look to her for the companionship and friendship that a normal man would find in relationships with other men. Or he may seek the affection, the uncritical acceptance and the guidance that a child needs from its mother. Both these relationships can be used to help him. His doctor will usually have full discussions with the ward team over the attitude he thinks each member should adopt towards the patient.

For a woman who is a homosexual the situation is reversed. Although she may be sexually attracted towards the female nurses she will look for friendship and comradeship to the male nurses and will regard them as she would her brother or her father.

Putting a male homosexual into a male ward is like putting a normal man into a women's ward. Perhaps both male and female homosexuals are best nursed in wards where patients and staff are mixed, or at least in wards where there are both men and women nurses. Remember that a male homosexual may try to get a male nurse on his own in order to make sexual advances to him. A female homosexual may do the same with a female nurse. Be aware of this possibility and arrange things so that, although you may be alone at times with such a patient, you are not completely out of sight of other people. This is wise both for the patient's sake and for your own.

All patients suffering from sexual disorder need to find as much self-expression and satisfaction as they can through leisure activities and relationships with other people.

Such a patient can sometimes develop latent talents and discover new interests through occupational therapy, and you can help by encouraging him to explore this to the full. Painting, modelling, pottery, carving, all forms of craft work, music, drama, dancing—any of these may offer a new outlet for him.

Similarly, it will be helpful if you can encourage him in any normal, creative relationship with other people. Use what ability he may have for organization and leadership by getting him actively involved in arranging social events, both in the ward itself and in the hospital as a whole. He may make a good ward representative on the patients' inter-ward committee.

Do not try to give these people advice, or point out what you may consider to be the error of their ways. They have given themselves all the advice in the world already. As for mending their ways, you might as well chide a lame man for not walking properly.

Let them talk to you if they can. There are few people outside hospital who are willing to listen to the problems of a sexual deviant, although there are many prepared to tell him what they think he should do. He may not feel able to talk to anyone except his doctor, but if he does want to talk to you keep your own opinions out of the way and concentrate on listening and helping him to go on talking. When he gets stuck don't jump in with 'Well, of course, *I* always say . . .'. It won't help him. Say instead 'What happened then?' or 'How did you feel about that?', or simply 'Yes?' with a rising note in your voice. This will help him to get going again. Very often the best that anyone can do for these people is to help them to make a more positive adjustment to their difficulties than they have been able to do so far. Only they can make the adjustment. They have to work it out for themselves. But we can sometimes offer the 'listening ear', and talking about a problem to a sympathetic listener can be a great help at times.

As with all patients, it is important that you keep an accurate record of what the patient says, what he does, and how he looks. His conversations with you and with other patients, any changes in his behaviour, the people he makes friends with, his dress and general appearance, whether he seems depressed or happier, anxious or relaxed, all should be entered carefully and frequently in the Nurses' Notes, for the information of his doctor and the rest of the ward team.

14

Looking after old people

The majority of patients in a psychiatric hospital are over sixty years of age.

Some of them are suffering from senile dementia, the mental illness associated with the wearing out of the brain in old age. Others have been in and out of hospital over the years, with recurrent attacks of depression or schizophrenia. A great many of them have simply grown old in hospital. They may have been admitted twenty or more years ago, with a mental illness. The illness became chronic and when the symptoms had subsided sufficiently for the patient to go home there was no longer any home to go to. Sons and daughters had married, husbands and wives had died or moved away and lost touch. There was no place any more for the patient in the outside community and no one who was willing to make a home for him. So he remained in hospital.

The modern concept of rehabilitation, which starts from the moment the patient enters hospital, is aimed at keeping him in touch with friends and relatives, preventing chronic illness and returning him to life outside hospital at the earliest moment, so that in the future the number of patients growing old in hospital should fall sharply.

Some people who are admitted to hospital when they are already old may not recover sufficiently to go home again, but a great many do and the same positive attitude towards rehabilitation is needed in geriatric wards as in the rest of the hospital.

The nursing of most old people in a psychiatric hospital is governed more by the infirmities of old age than by the symptoms of individual mental illnesses. Although with some the mental symptoms predominate, with most patients they tend to become blurred and overlaid by the characteristics common to all of us when our mental and physical powers begin to fail. Much physical care is necessary, work and leisure need thoughtful planning and personal relationships are as important for these people as for any other group of patients.

PHYSICAL CARE

The first thing to consider is how to keep old people out of bed and on their feet.

Once they take to staying in bed, they are liable to develop physical illnesses, particularly pneumonia, because they are inactive. Life becomes narrow and meaningless and they soon sink into a vegetable type of existence from which it is difficult, if not impossible, to rescue them.

Demented old people will need the same degree of help over personal hygiene, dressing and feeding as do regressed long-stay patients. Others may be able to look after themselves for the most part if you allow them plenty of time. The help you give will vary with each patient's particular difficulties. One will be able to dress himself but you may find he cannot do his shoe laces up. Another may not be able to raise her arms high enough to do her hair properly.

Most old people wake early and are quite happy to get up early, so there is no need for the morning routine to be rushed. It is essential that they should go at their own pace if they are to remain independent. Let them do all they possibly can for themselves and give them plenty of time in which to do it, but be close at hand to help where necessary.

Eyes, ears, teeth, hands and feet, bladder and bowels, are important for old people. If these are working well they can do much, but without them they may be lost, so get into the way of watching these points in every patient.

Eyes and ears

Look at what a patient cannot do and consider if it could be because he cannot see or hear properly.

Perhaps he is not interested in reading the newspaper or watching television. He seems clumsy and knocks little things over when he tries to pick them up. He doesn't answer when someone speaks to him, or complains that people are whispering about him. He doesn't want to join in games or attend entertainments. There may be other reasons for his behaviour, but it could all be explained by failing sight and hearing.

If you suspect that this is the cause let charge nurse know so that he can be fitted with spectacles or a hearing-aid if necessary. Neglected wax can also cause temporary deafness and is easily dealt with once it is noticed.

If he already has spectacles or a hearing aid see that they are plainly marked with his name and that he uses them all the time. If he keeps putting them on one side they probably need adjusting. It is worth paying a lot of attention to this because it will make life so much easier for him.

Teeth

Most patients will have dentures. See that they fit properly and that the patients use them. If a patient consistently takes his dentures out it may well be that they hurt him. It is no good expecting an old person to tell you this. Some may do so, but many will not. You must try to work out the reason for his behaviour yourself. Don't let him go on eating sloppy food. Try to find out what is wrong and let sister know, so that an appointment can be made for him to see the dentist if necessary.

Hands

Many old people are restless. They wander about touching this and that, they hoard rubbish, scratch their heads and rub their noses, they are absent-minded about personal hygiene and some are incontinent. Hands can easily carry infection in these circumstances. Pay extra attention to an old person's nails and skin. Keep the nails short and clean and see that the cuticles are not allowed to crack or tear.

Eating, washing, dressing, writing, in fact a dozen daily activities become difficult if fingers and wrists are stiff with arthritis or rheumatism. Wax baths are helpful but not always available. You can often do a lot with warm olive oil. Stand a small bottle of oil in a little hot water until it is thoroughly warmed. Pour a teaspoonful into your palm and massage the patient's hands for five minutes each day. You only need enough oil to make your hands move easily over his. Too much spoils the effect. Move his wrists and fingers and knead the backs of his hands and his palms firmly, doing one hand at a time. When you have finished wipe off any surplus oil with paper tissues, leaving a thin film to nourish the skin. Done regularly this can have an effect quite out of proportion to the small effort involved.

Feet

Most old people have trouble with their feet. Bunions, callouses, corns, horny or ingrowing toe nails, crossed toes, all make walking painful. Yet so much can be put right by a few visits to the chiropodist, and charge nurse or sister can easily arrange this once you let her know that it is necessary. See too that shoes fit properly, are wide enough across the toes and are not run down at the heel. If an old person is ready on his feet and can walk well it may mean all the difference between being bedfast or being up and about.

Bladder and bowels

Old people easily get constipated. Try to keep a check on their bowel movements and remember that diarrhoea can be a sign of chronic constipation.

If a newly admitted patient tells you he has taken a certain laxative regularly for a long time tell charge nurse about it. Sometimes it is unwise to break a habit which has been built up over a number of years. Fruit, vegetables, plenty of fluids and daily exercise will do much to establish normal bowel movements, but people with chronic constipation may need suppositories or an enema at first.

Watch also for the frequent passing of urine. In an old man this may be the first sign of an enlarged prostate.

Properly functioning bowels and bladder add so much to an old person's dignity and security. Many of his vague aches and pains may disappear if you can help him to overcome constipation and incontinence.

Bathing

Old people are often frightened of having a bath. A rubber mat in the bath helps to prevent slipping. Handles on the sides of the bath give a grip to help them pull themselves up. For those who find it difficult to sit down in the bath a small seat can be fixed, like a low-slung soap rack. Some find showers easier and these are fitted in many hospitals, but quite a lot of old people are afraid of them and prefer a seat in an ordinary bath.

Bath time is an excellent opportunity to take stock of a patient's physical condition and make mental notes of points which need attention, so while you help him to wash examine him carefully, from head to foot.

Meal times

Food means a lot to old people. For some it is practically the only real pleasure left to them, so try to make meal times as leisurely and enjoyable as you can.

See that patients are seated comfortably. Chairs should be high enough for them to reach their food without having to lift their elbows up. Raise them on cushions if you cannot change the chairs. See too that they are pushed up to the table so that they can sit at ease without leaning forward all the time.

Some will need their food cutting up because they cannot grip a knife and fork well enough to do it for themselves, but this can sometimes be overcome by padding the handles with foam rubber, or fitting handlebar grips to them. This can usually be done in the occupational therapy department. Plates with a plastic guard so that food cannot be pushed off are also useful for some patients.

Minced, sieved and soft food is easy to eat, but old people can manage other foods as well most of the time. What causes them difficulty is food which needs tearing or chewing for a long time. Tough pieces of meat are especially troublesome to them because they haven't the necessary strength in their jaws. Fish bones are difficult because they cannot see them, but filleted fish, haddock, cod, or boned herrings and kippers they can enjoy.

Nuts and any fruit which has pips or small hard pieces in it, such as raspberries, tomatoes, gooseberries, or currants, will be refused by people with dentures because the pips get between the plate and the roof of the mouth, which is painful and embarrassing. A few may be able to manage raw apples, oranges or pears on their own. Others can eat apple if it is sliced or grated and some will enjoy raw plums. Most of them will find bananas quite easy and squeezed orange juice sweetened with glucose will probably be enjoyed by everyone.

To help in the campaign against constipation include as many helpings of fruit and vegetables in their meals as you can, but you may find they take better to cooked fruit than to fresh.

The doctor may want a few patients to have special diets, for example, a reducing diet or a salt-free diet. You will have to see that these patients do not take sugar or salt, but most old people need their food to be well seasoned and sweetened if they are to enjoy it. Their taste buds are not as sensitive as those of younger people. It is better that they relish well-peppered meat and vegetables than refuse to eat because, to them, the food is insipid.

Serve small helpings and see that the slow eaters are started first. As with other patients, some will hoard food, some will eat their neighbour's share as well as their own and some may be liable to choke. You will have to guard against these tendencies and give extra attention when necessary.

Exercise

Exercise is vitally important to old people. It cannot be emphasized too strongly that daily, gentle exercise is essential in keeping them active. Walking in the open air is the best kind, not only because walking is gentle and the fresh air is good, but because it takes them out of the ward. There is something different to see, something to talk about when they get back. For a little while their world gets big again.

Old people can usually withstand as much bad weather as anyone else if they are warmly clothed and have good shoes. Probably the only conditions which need keep them indoors all day are fog or icy pavements.

Getting out of the hospital grounds, of course, is best of all, but even ten minutes walking round the ward garden every day can bring a more alert look and improved appetites. It is well worth helping patients to get dressed for literally ten minutes' walk, if that is all the weather or the staffing situation will allow. A few minutes every day will bring more benefit than an hour once a week.

HAZARDS FOR OLD PEOPLE

Stairs

Ideally old people should be nursed on the ground floor but this is not always possible because of the large numbers involved. Ground floor geriatric wards are usually reserved for those who cannot climb stairs. If you work in an upstairs ward be careful how you take patients up and down stairs. Give them plenty of time and pause on the landings to let them get their breath.

It is best to walk in front of a patient when going down stairs and behind him when coming up. If he stumbles you are then in the right position to stop him falling down the flight. See that the lights are switched on if it is at all dim and report at once any which are faulty. If you find one of the patients is having difficulty in getting up and down stairs let charge nurse know because it may be possible to arrange a transfer to the ground floor.

Fires

See that fires of all kinds are properly guarded. Try to stop patients getting lights for cigarettes by pushing slips of paper into the fire. Know where the fire extinguishers are and how they work. Learn the fire drill routine for your hospital.

If a patient's clothes catch fire lay him flat on the floor and wrap a rug or blanket round him to smother the flames.

Boiling water

Don't let frail old people carry heavy teapots or jugs

full of hot water. If there is an urn or water heater in the ward kitchen see that there is a stand underneath the tap. An accident can be caused by someone trying to hold a teapot full of boiling water with one hand while he turns off the tap with the other.

Hot-water bottles

People get less sensitive to heat and cold as they grow older. If hot-water bottles are used in your ward take every care to see that they are well protected. It is alarmingly easy to burn an old person.

Polished floors

Polish should never be used on the floors of geriatric wards because it is so easy for patients who are already unsteady on their feet to slip. Old bones are brittle and a fall may mean a broken leg. Most hospitals have a special seal applied to the floors which protects them and gives a long-lasting, non-slip shine.

Worn carpets

If you notice threadbare patches in carpets report them at once. Patients, and staff, may catch their heels and fall if these are not mended in the early stages.

Heights

See that patients do not climb on chairs or use steps, for example to get something down from the top shelf of a cupboard.

It is harder to get down than to climb up, as children and kittens soon learn. Also, if old people stand with their heads bent back for a few minutes, as they would while reaching up to get something, they often feel dizzy when they straighten their necks again. The head bent back has temporarily restricted the blood flow to the brain. If they are standing on a chair at the time they may fall and injure themselves.

SLEEP

Old people rarely sleep soundly all through the night. If they have a good rest after their midday meal they need not go to bed too early and this will give them a better chance of sleeping well.

Restricting drinks in the evening will mean that sleep is less likely to be disturbed by the need to go to the lavatory.

There will always be some who need sedation at night, but the night nurse should do all she can to help old people to sleep without drugs. Attention to the patient's comfort (see Chapter Nine) will often succeed in helping him to get off to sleep. Some old people are frightened of the dark and will sleep better if the light is left on.

Drugs given at night so often leave a patient heavy and apathetic, or slightly confused the next day. This means he does not share fully in the day's activities and only recovers in the evening. At bedtime he doesn't feel like going to sleep, is given more sedation, and so a vicious circle is set up.

WORK AND LEISURE

Old people need a pattern of work and recreation to their day like everyone else, but the work time needs to be shorter and the rests more frequent. Both work and recreation must be simple and not tiring, either physically or mentally.

Often the ordinary housekeeping of the ward will provide enough for them. They can make beds, lay tables, help with clearing away and washing up, sweep, dust, polish furniture, arrange flowers, or do simple mending. Sometimes the industrial therapy unit will have a simple piece of work they can do, or the occupational therapy department may be able to provide materials for Christmas decorations, cross-stitch cushion covers, rag rugs, cane baskets, knitting or scrap books. Whatever the task is it is important to see that they do not tire themselves, and you should always be on the watch for this.

Many of them may enjoy card games and it helps if you learn to play so that you can join in with them. Women may like playing the piano, or making little cakes for tea. Men like dominoes, ludo, cribbage, draughts, or shove ha'penny, and everyone can help with a jigsaw. Put it on a large tray so that it can be lifted off intact whenever the table is needed for something else.

Pets are often popular. Budgerigars, hamsters, rabbits, guinea pigs, tortoises, goldfish, all provide something to watch and care for. In the summer a piece of the garden can be used to grow lettuce, radishes and cress. Cress can also be grown indoors in winter on a windowsill and a row of orange and apple pips, labelled with patients' names, can be a source of interest.

Community singing of the old-time songs and marches goes well and so does a programme of records in which patients can have their own requests played. Sometimes the patients themselves, with the help of the occupational therapists and the nurses, can form a band, supplying the rhythm on drums, cymbals and triangle, while someone plays the melody on the piano.

PERSONAL RELATIONSHIPS

Old people are not easy to nurse. Many are obstinate, suspicious, greedy and quarrelsome. Others are foolish, uninhibited, dirty and full of self-pity. Those who have grown old in the hospital may be relatively stable, but demented patients and those who have recently been admitted can be a difficult nursing problem. Many are depressed and show this by delusions of guilt and preoccupation with their bowels and digestion.

Yet a skilled nurse can often achieve a surprising improvement in an old person. Try not to lose your temper with him. Remind yourself that his behaviour is the result of illness, not malice. Never hurry old people. It is unkind and it is also a waste of time, because so often when they are hurried they become confused and the task takes twice as long after all. Keep to a simple routine and don't change it. These patients cannot adjust to new ways or new ideas.

Most of them will have likes and dislikes which may seem petty to onlookers but mean a lot to the patient himself. Consider carefully before you insist on them giving these up. Do they really matter so much? If Mr A has always had jam with his bacon it won't poison him now. If Mrs B likes to take that dreadful old carrier bag with her wherever she goes and even likes to sit on it at mealtimes it doesn't really do her, or anyone else, any harm. If you try to alter these habits you may simply achieve an agitated, resentful patient. Try to go along with the little things so that you can be firm over the big things, like dressing properly, washing, taking exercise, persevering with spectacles or hearing aid, eating adequate meals and writing home regularly.

If a patient hoards rubbish try to come to an agreement with him, for example, that he will keep it in a certain place and in return for non-interference during the week he will let you have a turn out every Saturday.

Try not to patronize old people by calling them 'Gran' or 'Dad'. Bus conductors and shop assistants do this as a sign of affection and goodwill towards old people. They have no time, nor is the situation appropriate, to ask the person's proper name. But a nurse who does it is really saying that although she knows the patient's name she can't be bothered to use it. She wouldn't call the senior nursing officer 'Dad', and she should not allow herself to justify it with Mr B because he's 'only a patient'.

Nurses defend this practice by saying that patients

like it, but this is rarely so. If you ask patients the
majority say they prefer to be addressed by their names.
The same holds good for the use of Christian names with
old people. A few may genuinely like the nurses to call
them 'Rosie' or 'Bill', others have become so accustomed
to it over the years that they hardly notice, or are too
apathetic to protest in any case, but others actively
resent it, especially from nurses young enough to be their
grandchildren.

Relatives often feel guilty when an old person has to
come into hospital. When they come to see him try to
make them feel they did the right thing, that they are
partners with the nurses and doctors in caring for him.
Encourage patients to write to friends and relatives each
week and help them to do so if necessary.

Perhaps more than anything else old people want
someone who will talk with them. Try to find some time
every day when you can sit down with a group of patients
and just chat. Most of them have little recollection of
what was in yesterday's paper, but they can often remember vividly what happened fifty years ago and
they love to reminisce. Let them go over old memories,
compare notes and cap each others' stories—school-
days, holidays, courting, the war—they all remember
these.

The thought of death distresses some patients and they
may speak about it to you. If you have come to terms
with this thought yourself you will be able to help them,
but if not don't change the subject too quickly. Help
them to talk if they can. Just saying their thoughts aloud
to a sympathetic listener can be a relief and you may
learn of some practical problem, such as provision for a
wife or child, which is worrying them. If this happens let
charge nurse know because often something can be done
to ease their minds. The social worker may be able to help.
The chaplain too is always ready to visit patients who need
him. He works closely with the doctors and nurses, and

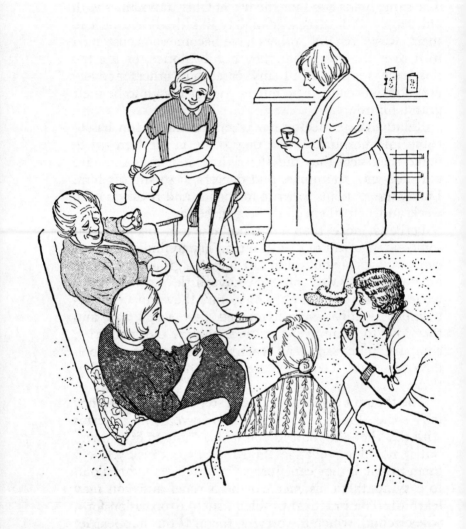

can often bring peace and comfort when other methods have failed.

For the generation which is now in its seventies one of the pleasantest times of the day used to be tea time. Married women rarely went out to work before the 1914 war. Tea time meant a gathering of the family after the business of the day. The children came in from school and the husband came home from the factory or the office. The curtains were drawn and the kettle was put on. There was no television, the cinema was in its infancy and only a handful of people had a radio. The family provided its own entertainment for the rest of the evening. Try, if you can, to recapture for them a little of the companionship that tea time meant. Let them sit by the fire, or dream in the sunshine and recall some of their happier times.

The care of old people, in all its forms, is specialized work and the members of the team who can make the biggest contribution to their progress are often the nursing staff. By paying constant attention to an old person's physical health, keeping him active and occupied and helping him to find companionship you will often achieve worthwhile improvements.

15

Children and adolescents

A happy, normal childhood is the best preparation for adult life, but unfortunately not all children have this advantage. For some of them childhood and adolescence bring so much stress that psychiatric help becomes necessary.

A child may have parents who did not want him, to whom he is just a nuisance, something that gets in the way of what they want to do. Perhaps his parents dislike one another and the home is full of their nagging hostility. Sometimes a mother's love is so possessive that the child lives, as it were, in a hot-house and shrivels up when he meets the cool air outside. Other parents are so strict and narrow that their children become emotionally stunted, unable to respond normally to life's opportunities. Some parents reject a child because he has a physical handicap such as epilepsy or brain damage, or they become over-protective and communicate their fears to him so that he grows up in an atmosphere of constant anxiety.

In these situations the relationship between the child and his parents is full of pain and unhappiness. Some children manage to grow up normally in spite of this, but for others the strain is too great and they become emotionally disturbed.

As a rule children are not able to describe their feelings

in so many words, but they show that they are disturbed by the way they behave. The following are examples of behaviour which indicates that a child is disturbed.

Stealing	Telling lies
Nightmares	Bed wetting
Playing truant	Stammering
Nail biting	Temper tantrums

Some young children withdraw completely from the world around them. They stop speaking and seem unaware of other people. They do not join in other children's games and seem not to know how to play. All communication between them and the rest of the world seems to have broken down. This kind of behaviour is described as autistic.

Adolescence is a time of great upheaval for a young person. If, in addition, he has an unsatisfactory relationship with his parents he also may find the strain too much. Adolescents sometimes develop mental illnesses as adults do, and may suffer from depression or schizophrenia or one of the neuroses. They may also show their disturbance by disordered behaviour, such as

Destructiveness	Cruelty
Fighting	Solitariness
Staying out at night	Sexual misdemeanours
Stealing	

Children and adolescents come to have psychiatric treatment in a variety of ways. Sometimes the parents, finding that they can no longer control the child, will ask for advice from their general practitioner and he will arrange for them either to have an appointment with the psychiatrist in the out-patient department of the local hospital, or to attend the child guidance clinic in their area. This is a clinic run by the local health authority at which the child can be seen by a doctor who specializes in child psychiatry. It may be that the school teacher notices the child's behaviour and draws the attention of the school doctor to him. Or it may only be when the child appears before a Juvenile Court that he is referred for treatment.

Many children and adolescents can be treated as out-patients, or in day hospitals, but some will need a period in hospital, either because their symptoms are too severe for them to be cared for adequately outside, or because it is necessary to separate them from their parents' influence for a while.

Those under twelve years of age are usually admitted to the children's ward while the adolescent ward takes those between thirteen and sixteen. From seventeen onwards they are admitted to the adult ward.

The ward routine is built round a framework of getting up, meal times, school work, interviews with the doctor, exercise, recreation and going to bed, but only the broad outlines are fixed because the patients' ages vary considerably and so do their needs, and the routine must be sufficiently flexible to suit them all.

Some children will need help or supervision when washing and dressing, others can look after themselves in this respect. Everyone who can do so is encouraged to help with the ward work, making beds, laying tables, and so on.

There will probably be a school in the hospital grounds and all the children who are well enough to do so will go to school for a few hours both morning and afternoon. The teachers in the school are not only qualified in teaching but are also experienced in helping disturbed children.

The rest of the day, apart from meal times and interviews with the doctor, will be spent in various forms of play and creative hobbies. Young children need a sand pit and a pool. Energetic boys and girls want an adventure playground, something to climb, something to jump off, something to crawl through, something to swing on and something to build with. Quieter children may like a blackboard and chalks, large sheets of paper with paints and crayons, or dolls and teddy bears. Adolescents need to be able to make a noise. They will want space and opportunities for physical exercise.

The occupational therapist can offer a whole range of activities which will capture the children's interest: modelling, carpentry, puppets, dressmaking, fretwork, marquetry for the older ones, scrapbooks, a dolls' house, paper cutouts, raffia work, dressing up for the others. In addition, adolescents may enjoy athletics, dancing, team games and debates.

Coming into hospital can be a frightening experience for a child, whatever his age. Home may be an unhappy place, but at least he knows the unhappiness there and has worked out some way of hiding from it. What can he do to escape the new threat of hospital?

His parents too are distressed. Often they have genuinely tried to do their best for him and have no idea why things have gone wrong. They feel guilty, without knowing why, and are just as anxious about the child's admission as he is himself. A few parents will be glad to be rid of their children and may try to disguise this by an aggressively critical attitude towards you and the rest of the team.

When a child is admitted welcome him and his parents in a friendly way, but let them do the talking. The child needs to get used to you and the parents want to put their side of the story to you. Take them slowly round the ward and let them see everything—the other children and what they are doing, the dining-room, the play area, the dormitories. Give them plenty of time and answer as many of their questions as you can. If you are doubtful or do not know the answer, say so and refer the question to charge nurse. Be careful not to make promises unless you are certain you can keep them. Children take a promise quite literally and for most of these children life is already full of broken ones.

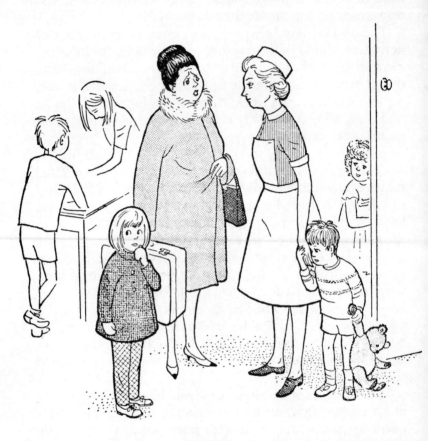

Coming into hospital can be a frightening experience for a child, and a friendly welcome for him and his parents, a walk round the ward to see other children at work and play, may help him to adjust to the new surroundings

The child may ask you something but he is more likely to be all eyes, taking everything in. Make a point of noticing what he does say and write it down, as soon as you can, in his Nurses' Notes. It will be helpful to his doctor.

The parents, on the other hand, may not only want to know where he will sleep, what time he will get up, and so on, they may also want to tell you how he should be looked after. He never eats apples, he likes brown sugar not white on his cornflakes, he easily gets a chill so he wears a woollen vest all the year round, and are the hospital sheets aired properly? The other children look a bit rough and he certainly mustn't be allowed to play on the shute like those boys over there, it's far too dangerous!

This is their way of saying they have done their best and it isn't really their fault. Be friendly and interested in what they tell you. Thank them for all the information they are giving you. Tell them how helpful it will be to you and to all the other members of the ward team. Let them see that you are sympathetic towards them, but avoid giving your own opinions or making definite statements about how their child will, or will not, be treated.

Helping the parents to modify their attitude towards the child may be as important as treating the child. Sometimes the mother and father are found to be even more in need of help than he is. For this reason the doctor and the social worker keep in close touch with the parents throughout the child's stay in hospital, having regular interviews with them and helping them to prepare for the child's return home.

For the time that the child is in hospital the ward becomes his home. He will look on the nurses as his parents and will behave towards them in much the same way as he does towards his mother and father.

All children and adolescents need affection, approval and guidance. A child is not happy when there are no rules and he is allowed to do exactly as he pleases. He wants to know what the rules are and to be sure that they are applied fairly. He wants to know that your affection for him is real, that it will go on even if he is disobedient, and that you truly are on his side.

At first he may be quiet and do whatever you tell him, but sooner or later he will feel compelled to test you out by defiance or disobedience. When this happens let him see that you do not approve of his behaviour, but keep the same friendly attitude towards him that you have always had. If he refuses to come in to tea at the right time he will not be able to go swimming with the others tomorrow. Tell him you are sorry about this, but he knows the rule as well as you do. This is just, and both he and the other children can see that it is so. But don't later in the day refuse to let him do his usual job of helping you with the evening drinks, and when you tuck the children in bed and go round saying goodnight don't leave him out 'because he was a naughty boy this afternoon'. Treat him just as you always have done. When tomorrow comes be quite matter of fact about the swimming. It's a pity, but there it is, he'll have to stay behind today.

In this way he will learn that you approve of him as a person, that you like him, although you may disapprove of his behaviour. This will help him to conform to the rules and to want to behave in an acceptable way. If you reject him and he feels you are no longer interested in him he may be driven to more and more defiance in an effort to regain your attention.

Disturbed children need a chance to work out their problems in a calm atmosphere. They cannot talk about what hurts them so they act it out in the way they behave. Nightmares, temper tantrums, fighting, disobedience, withdrawal, are all ways of showing their anxiety.

Much of your work in these wards will be playing with groups of children and keeping them happily occupied.

It is important that you should join in the game and not simply stand and watch, because then you will be able to influence the children more easily. Watch for the child who is always on the edge of the group and needs to be gently encouraged to join in. Try to anticipate the one who feels he is not getting enough attention and may start fighting if you do not create a diversion. If a child has a temper tantrum sit quietly beside him until he is calm again. Remember that this is his way of saying that he feels dreadful and can't stand it any more. Never be angry with him, or shut him in a room by himself. This will only increase his anxiety and therefore make his behaviour worse.

Disturbed children can be exasperating, but try not to show your irritation or lose your temper. If you can keep a calm, consistent attitude towards them they will begin to feel more secure in their relationships with all adults and will gradually be able to give up their disturbed behaviour. You will also find it much easier to control them if you remain quietly confident.

Since most of the children cannot describe their feelings easily the doctor will depend a great deal on your reports of the way they play and how they behave towards the nurses and towards each other. As a rule each nurse is given several children about whom she will write frequent notes. Try to describe their play in as much detail as you can and notice particularly what situations cause them to become upset.

Both children and adolescents form close relationships with the nursing staff. Each has his own favourite nurse. To a large extent your group will copy what you do and tend to adopt your attitudes and your way of thinking. This means that they can be influenced quite considerably through you and your relationship with them can be used to help their progress. The sharing of information among the various members of the ward team is most important if this is to be successful, and there will be frequent staff meetings to discuss how each patient should be treated.

In this situation it is easy to become attached to the young people you are trying to help and to be distressed when the time comes for them to go home. This is natural, but try to remember that you are only temporarily taking the place of the parent. If you become dependent on their attachment to you, you can no longer help them. Far from being sad that you are losing them, you should be thinking of how best to ease the parting for them, so that they can leave hospital with the least possible disturbance and continue to make progress back into the community.

16

Talking with patients

When the patient has an interview with his doctor they sit down together and the patient tries to tell the doctor about his problems. The doctor is interested and wants to help the patient. The patient becomes aware of this. Gradually he begins to trust his doctor and have confidence in him. Because the patient talks to him, trusts him and has confidence in him, the doctor may be able to help the patient to find some solution to his problems. Using the relationship between them in this way is called psychotherapy.

With one patient the doctor will concentrate on simply relieving his symptoms and helping him to adjust to his present situation. This is supportive psychotherapy.

With another he may try to make him realize the underlying causes of his distress. To do this he helps him to recall memories of painful experiences in his early life which he has repressed, and then to find a better way of dealing with them. This is analytical psychotherapy.

PSYCHOANALYSIS

Psychoanalysis is an intense form of analytical psycho-therapy in which the doctor meets the patient almost every day over a period of several years. It is suitable for only a few patients and is too time-consuming to be used to any extent in a hospital.

The principles of psychoanalysis were laid down by Dr Freud in 1900. The names of Dr Jung and Dr Adler, who followed him, are associated with variations of the basic Freudian analysis.

GROUP PSYCHOTHERAPY

Sometimes the doctor will treat several patients together in a group. He may use supportive psychotherapy with one group and more analytical methods with another, depending on the kind of difficulties the patients are facing.

Through group psychotherapy the doctor can give more of his time to the patients than he could if he saw them all individually. A group of six to ten patients will meet regularly with the doctor and will discuss their problems with him, and with each other.

When a patient first becomes a member of a group like this he may feel too self-conscious or too embarrassed to speak, but after a time, as he listens to the others, he begins to see that he is not as alone as he thought. Others have their doubts, their worries, anxieties and weaknesses, not unlike his own. They too feel guilty, depressed, mixed up, or angry, just as he does. Sometimes, as they and the doctor talk together, he finds he can see a little of what went wrong in their lives. He begins to understand why they have become the sort of people they are today.

As he gets to feel more at home in the group he starts, haltingly at first, but with increasing confidence, to tell them some of his own difficulties. They and the doctor listen with interest. The patients sympathise, make comments and offer advice. The doctor may ask a question, or point out a similar situation in another patient's story. The patient comes to realise that he reacts to certain situations in the same way, time and time again. Gradually he discerns a pattern in his life, and as he previously saw what had gone wrong in other patients' lives, he now begins to see what has gone wrong in his own.

When he can see how his past experiences are influencing his present behaviour he is gaining insight. Once the patient has some insight into the causes of his difficulties he may be helped either to resolve them, or to make a more constructive adjustment to them, and this is the aim of both group and individual psychotherapy.

BEHAVIOUR THERAPY

When you are training your dog to wait at the kerb before crossing the road you reward him with a pat and a word of praise when he obeys you, and you probably give him a smart tap and speak sharply to him when he disobeys. He comes to associate obedience with praise and affection, and disobedience with discomfort and disapproval. He wants your praise, so he learns to do the things which please you, and to avoid doing the things which anger you.

Human beings react in a similar way. As children we learn quickly from the teacher who gives us praise and affection. We also learn quickly to treat boiling kettles, penknives, stinging-nettles, and other potentially harmful objects, with respect, because we know that if we do not do so we shall get hurt.

Behaviour therapy makes use of this learning principle to change a patient's behaviour, and is often used in the treatment of isolated symptoms, when it may be unnecessary to subject him to intensive psychotherapy. Some patients have irrational fears, or phobias (see p. 108), such as a fear of open spaces, of cats or spiders, of heights, and so on, which greatly restrict them in their everyday lives, and many of these can be removed through behaviour therapy.

A woman became literally terrified of cats. She would sweat and tremble in panic if one came into the room, and she could not rest if she knew that one was anywhere in the house. She came to dread going out in case she should see a cat, and would go far out of her way to avoid this. Shopping became a nightmare, and even in her own house she was constantly on edge in case she should catch sight of a cat through the window.

In his interviews with her the doctor first helped her to relax, by giving her a suitable sedative. He then asked her to think, not of a cat, but of a photograph of a cat—just a piece of paper with a cat's face on it. Even to do this caused her severe distress, but with repeated encouragement and relaxation she did do so, and after a time he was able to place an actual photograph of a cat in the room. With more encouragement and praise for her efforts she brought herself to take the photograph in her hands and really look at it. In this way, a step at a time, she made headway, until after a few weeks she could even bear to stay in the same room with a live cat, and when she finally came to the end of the treatment she was able to pick up a cat and stroke it, like anyone else. Each step forward had weakened her fear, until its hold on her was broken and she learnt to replace it with more normal behaviour.

Such intense and irrational fears sometimes seem stupid, or even laughable, to people who have had no experience of them. It is important that nurses should understand how real they are to the patient, and should treat him accordingly. Trying to force such a patient beyond his ability to cope with the fear would simply undo all the good that was being done in his interviews with the doctor. The nurse's part in behaviour therapy is firstly to protect the patient from whatever it is that he fears in his environment. In the case of the woman who hated cats it would be necessary to see that no cats entered the ward, and that no pictures of cats, in magazines, newspapers, or in any other form, were seen by the patient until she was capable of facing them. Secondly, the nurse should do her best to enlist the sympathy of other patients for the phobic patient by assuring them that his fear is genuine, and she should demonstrate to them, by her own attitude towards the patient, that she takes his fears seriously. Thirdly, she should support and encourage him in every way as he tries to overcome his fear.

Aversion therapy is another form of behaviour therapy, in which the doctor tries to build up an association in the patient's mind between his behaviour and some form of unpleasant sensation. It is used to treat alcoholism (see p. 175) and sexual deviations. When he uses Antabuse to help a patient who is dependent on alcohol the doctor is trying to associate drink, in the patient's mind, with headache, nausea and severe physical distress, and the patient learns to avoid alcohol because of this association. The administration of an emetic, or of repeated small electric shocks, are other ways of producing an unpleasant association, and these are used in attempts to cure sexual deviations.

Behaviour therapy is often successful, but there are also times when the removal of the patient's symptom reveals an underlying illness which was not at first apparent, and which then requires much more prolonged and intensive treatment. For this reason not all doctors are in favour of it.

TRANSFERENCE

When a patient is having psychotherapy the relationship between him and his doctor becomes rather like that of a child with a parent. Often he will feel towards his doctor as he did in childhood towards his mother or father, or as he once did towards a teacher, an elder brother, or a girl friend. This is called transference, because the patient transfers to his doctor some of the feelings he had in childhood for these other people. It means that sometimes the patient will have warmth, admiration and trust for his doctor. At other times he will be angry, frightened, jealous, or hurt. All these feelings are used by the doctor in helping the patient to understand his difficulties.

THE NURSE-PATIENT RELATIONSHIP

Just as the relationship between the doctor and the patient is a therapeutic one, so is that between the nurse and the patient. Occasionally the nurse may be asked to play a specific role in a patient's psychotherapy, under the direction of the doctor in charge of his treatment, but more usually her contribution is to give support and encouragement to all patients, and to provide for them the understanding and accepting relationship which they have been unable to find in the world outside.

In a general hospital the nurse may give patients injections, dress wounds, help to put plasters on and take them off again, assist at surgical operations and operate complicated equipment in her efforts to help them recover. In a psychiatric hospital there is little nursing of this nature, except in the few wards set aside for people who are also physically ill. The complicated equipment that you will use as a psychiatric nurse is your own personality, and the way in which you will use it most frequently is by talking with patients.

All the time nurses and patients are together an interaction is going on between them, whether they are aware of it or not. The nurse who hardly says a word and goes round with a face like a wet suet pudding is having just as much effect on the patients as the nurse who is alive and interested and always has time to talk. The first nurse has a negative relationship with the patients and her attitude retards their recovery, while the second nurse has a positive relationship and her presence in the ward is therapeutic.

Broadly speaking, you should have five aims in mind when you are talking with patients.

1. To create a relationship of trust and confidence between you.
2. To help a patient put his problems into words.
3. To draw him back from his world of fantasy.
4. To reassure him and to relieve tension.
5. To help patients to talk to other people and make normal social contacts.

TRUST AND CONFIDENCE

Once you find that someone has told you a deliberate lie your confidence in that person is badly shaken. It may be a long time before you trust him again. It is the same with patients, so be truthful in what you say. It is not always helpful to tell the whole of the truth, but there is a lot of difference between giving a limited but truthful answer, and telling what you know to be a lie.

For example, Mr A's progress is much slower than everyone had hoped it would be. Mr A says 'Do you think I shall ever get any better, Nurse?' If you say 'Why, of course you will Mr A. You'll be out of here in no time!' you are telling him something which you know is untrue. Moreover, he will suspect that it is a lie and think that you just can't be bothered with him. On the other hand, if you say, 'Well, as a matter of fact Mr A we all expected you to do much better, and we're disappointed that you have made so little progress,' you will be telling the truth, but Mr A, to say the least, will not feel encouraged.

Try dealing with it along these lines

Mr A. 'Shall I ever get any better, Nurse?'
Nurse. 'Well, how do you feel, Mr A?'
Mr A. 'Oh, pretty much the same I think.'
Nurse. 'Let's see, what are you making in occupational therapy now?'
Mr A. 'A coffee table—I've nearly finished it.'

Nurse. 'You weren't doing that when you first went to O.T.'

Mr A. 'No. I was scraping those bedsteads.'

Nurse. 'And before that you just didn't do anything at all—I'd call that progress, you know.'

Mr A. (*brightening*). 'Well, I suppose I am a bit better really.'

Nurse. 'Come and give me a hand with the score cards for tonight.'

Look, not at how far he still has to go, but at how far he has come. Try to help him to see it for himself. Maybe his hallucinations are no better, but all the same you have been able to find something which is both true and encouraging. If you cannot find any sign of progress at all there is always hope, and you can tell the patient so. Many people have been known to show improvement when everyone had thought this was quite impossible.

If patients ask you a question to which you do not know the answer, say that you do not know, and suggest that they ask doctor or charge nurse. Never make up an answer to questions such as 'When shall I go home?' 'How many more shock treatments must I have?' 'Will this treatment cure me?' or 'Can I go on leave next week?'

Similarly, don't make promises unless you are reasonably certain that you can keep them. If you are forced to break your promise explain to the patient at the first opportunity, and say how sorry you are. To make a promise just to keep a patient quiet, when you have no intention of carrying it out, is both cruel and damaging to them.

Sometimes, of course, you will feel irritated by patients, perhaps depressed over their lack of progress, or anxious about their unpredictable behaviour. Try, in spite of your feelings, to keep a quiet, friendly attitude towards them. The more consistent your own behaviour is, the more confidence the patient will have in you. At the same time you are showing him, by your example, how

a mature person deals with the frùstrations and annoy-
ances of everyday living.

PATIENTS' PROBLEMS

One of the most important services you can offer the
patient is to help him to put his problems into words, and
you should always be looking for opportunities to encourage patients to talk.

Your part is not to talk *to* the patient, but to help him
to talk to you—or to other people.

Some of what he says may seem trivial and time-wast-
ing, other things may shock or startle you. If you turn
away from him he will either feel that you are not interested, or that he cannot risk talking to you freely. Try to
keep a noncommittal attitude.

At first you will find yourself searching round for
answers to his questions, or trying to find suitable comments when he makes a statement, but this will not help
him. If he needs guidance and advice his doctor is the
person to give it to him. Your part is to help him to look
at his problems. Learn to answer a question with a
question, and a statement by a repetition of the statement. This will make it easier for him to go on talking.

For example, if Mr A says 'I wish I could drive,' and
you say 'Oh, so do I! It must be fun to have a car,' this is
a friendly response, but the patient doesn't really want
to know whether you also would like to drive, and if you
reply like this the conversation may well stop there.

On the other hand, if you ask a question, 'What is it
you like about driving?' or 'Where would you go?' you
give him an invitation to elaborate on what he has just
said. If you repeat his statement, 'You would like to
drive?' he may go on 'Yes. I remember when I was at
school . . .'—and you now begin to get what was really
in his mind when he brought up the subject of driving.
This is what he wanted to talk about, but he didn't know

how to begin. Your part is to make it easier for him to begin, and to go on.

Try to guard against making hasty comments when you are startled. If Mr A says 'My wife hates me!' you may find yourself exclaiming 'Oh, I'm sure she doesn't Mr A!'—but this is not in the least helpful. Mr A may be perfectly right in thinking that Mrs A hates him. In any case your words are a rebuff—you have turned away from him in your mind, even if you are still sitting beside him. Again, learn to ask a question or repeat his statement as a question. 'What makes you think that, Mr A?' or 'She hates you?' In either case your reply invites a further response from Mr A.

Avoid asking 'Why?' This question may be a little frightening to a patient. It can be disconcerting to be asked, point blank, 'Why did you do that?' Try it out on your friends and notice their reaction. 'What made you do that?' is a more gentle inquiry.

The important thing is that the patient should ventilate his problems. Your contribution is to help him to do so by making it as easy as possible, and to share what he says with the rest of the team—not to give advice, or to make judgements.

Sometimes the patient may say that he doesn't want anyone else to know what he has told you. Tell him that the doctor should know about it because it will be useful to him in his efforts to help the patient. Offer to tell the doctor for him. Many patients will agree to this.

If he is not willing for you to tell the doctor try to persuade him to do so himself. Do not break his confidence by reporting what he has said in spite of his request for secrecy, but tell charge nurse that you are trying to persuade him to confide in his doctor about something he has told you. Continue your efforts whenever there is an opportunity.

You may find, after a while, that another member of the staff reports the same thing. Some patients talk to several people on the same topic 'in confidence' because they are seeking extra attention. Don't take this personally, it is part of the patient's illness. Meet it by trying to give him attention in more acceptable ways.

There is one exception to what has been said above. If what the patient tells you indicates that he is thinking of injuring himself, or someone else, and he says it is in confidence, explain to him that although in every other instance you would respect his confidence, when it is a question of his own or another person's safety you have an absolute duty to report it. Go immediately to charge nurse or sister and tell her what he has said, no matter what protest he makes. If possible get the patient to go with you.

DELUSIONS AND HALLUCINATIONS

A patient's delusions and hallucinations are perfectly real to him. If you argue about them you simply convince him that you do not understand. But a careful explanation of what is going on around him may sometimes help to reduce them.

To a deluded patient the many comings and goings in the ward often have a sinister significance and relate directly to unpleasant things which he believes are about to happen to him. Frequently the ward is thought to be a charade, designed to cloak the activities of some organization which is out to harm him, or bring him the punishment he knows he deserves. Avoid reference to his delusions or hallucinations, but go out of your way to tell him what you, and other members of the staff, are doing. Not only once, but all through the day, whenever you think of it. Without this explanation he may misinterpret the simplest activities and take them to be confirmation of his delusions.

If charge nurse or his doctor asks you to find out more about his hallucinations you can say, for example, 'These voices you say you can hear—what do they talk **about**?' or with a visual hallucination, 'No, I can't see it, but how does it seem to you?' This avoids unprofitable argument without reinforcing the patient's conviction.

In talking with a deluded patient try to discover the areas of his personality which are untouched by the delusions and develop these. For example, a patient may be convinced that the end of the world is at hand, yet show a lively interest in the next season's fashions, or insist that his legs are made of putty, yet be an accomplished dancer. Under these circumstances forget about the end of the world, bring out the sewing machine and the record player, and talk about the latest patterns and the hit parade.

REASSURANCE AND RELIEF OF TENSION

As you come to know the patients in your ward better you will sometimes be able to see when they are becoming anxious or tense by the way they look and behave. If you draw them into conversation with you they may find relief through talking and you may prevent an aggressive outburst.

If a patient does start behaving aggressively, for instance, throwing things about or threatening other people, one of you should remain with the rest of the patients, one remove any broken objects, and a third attempt to calm the patient.

Remember that aggressive people are frightened people. They are afraid that if they do not attack something dreadful will happen. By being aggressive they are warding off danger. When we are frightened we easily misunderstand what people do and say, so your first objective will be to make it quite plain to the patient that you intend him no harm. If he is injuring himself or someone else you will have to move quickly and stop him, but if for instance he has torn up a pile of magazines and thrown them over the floor, or flung his cup and saucer at the wall, take your time.

Walk slowly towards him. If you move quickly he may think you are going to attack him. This will make him more frightened, and therefore more aggressive. Hold your hands open, with the palms turned towards him, either at your sides or in front of you, so that he can see you are not holding anything.

Speak in a low, quiet voice as you approach him. Ask him what is upsetting him and suggest that he might like to tell you about it. Do not attempt to touch him, or to go right up to him at first, in case he thinks you are trying to make a grab at him. Tell him that you want to help him. If he goes on shouting, continue to speak quietly to him, repeating your wish to help and your suggestion that he should talk to you about what is troubling him.

Be as relaxed as you can while you do this. Take a deep breath and deliberately let your muscles go slack. This is important, because your reaction gets over to the patient. If you are tense he will remain aggressive. If you are relaxed he will begin to relax also.

When you see this happening, sit down and invite him to sit beside you. In this way you let him approach you. He will feel safer like this. Once seated, listen, and try to find out what started the outburst. Talking about it will help him to calm down and may throw some light on how such behaviour can be prevented in the future. Whatever he tells you should be reported in his notes and, of course, to charge nurse and the rest of the ward team.

Sometimes a patient behaves in a disturbed way because he is confused and doesn't know who he is, or what is happening. In this case you must tell him his name, your name, and where he is, over and over if necessary, until he begins to grasp it.

'Mr A, you are in X hospital, and I am Nurse Z.' Say this clearly and quietly. Look directly at him and try to

221

get him to look at you. Tell him that he is safe here and that you will prevent any harm coming to him. If he wanders about go with him, so that you are always close beside him. Ask him questions to see if he has understood what you have said. When he is quieter get him to sit down with you and try, by listening, to find out as much about the incident as you can.

TALKING WITH A GROUP

Mentally ill people often find difficulty in mixing with others. An important part of your work is helping them to talk to one another.

Whenever you have a group of patients together, with time to spare, start them talking. Choose a subject that is likely to be of general interest, but not too serious. If you pick up a magazine you will have plenty of ideas straight away. Introduce it casually—'I say! Look at this,' and pass the magazine around. When someone makes a response take up what he says and use it, even if it is not directly connected with the topic you chose. The subject doesn't matter. What you want is to get them talking.

Remember your technique of asking a question or repeating a statement. If you pass round a picture of a holiday resort and Mr A says, 'I've been there', don't say 'So have I. We went there last June. I think it's such a pretty place and the sands are wonderful.' If you go on like this you will find when you stop that the patients are either sitting silently, waiting for you to start again, or have wandered away into their own private worlds and are paying no attention. Instead, take up Mr A's remark and help him to say more. 'You've been there Mr A?' or 'What did you think of it?' and so on.

As soon as someone joins in, help him in the same way and keep the talk going between them. When several people are talking you will be able to join in a little more yourself, but remember your purpose. You are not, on this occasion, aiming to talk *to* patients. At another time this could be a useful thing to do, for instance when you want to give them some information, but with the present group your aim is to help them to talk to each other, to come out of their separate worlds and meet each other on common ground.

Notice the people who don't talk and try to bring them in, but be careful how you do it. If you know for example that Mr B, who has said nothing, is keen on sailing, steer the conversation towards this topic to give him an opening. 'I wonder if there's much sailing at that place you went to Mr A?' Don't address Mr B personally. It can be frightening to be picked out by name in front of a group of people. At first Mr B may just nod or say 'Yes' in agreement with something another patient has said. This is a beginning. It means he is reaching out. When he does manage a sentence take it up straight away so that he can go on.

The safest way is simply to repeat what he has said. Even a related question at this stage may be too much for him. For example, Mr B finally mumbles something about '. . . tide very strong down there'. If you say, 'How much sailing have you done Mr B?' or 'Why is the tide so strong?' he is more likely to relapse into silence again than if you simply say 'The tide's very strong?' Notice that 'Why?' and 'How?' are very direct questions, which can sometimes give a person the feeling that he is being challenged.

Once you have helped Mr B to say a few sentences don't press him any further for a while, but keep him and all the quiet ones in mind, and draw them in from time to time.

Notice that you sometimes get just 'Yes' and 'No' in answer to your questions and the conversation is then in danger of coming to a standstill. This is because you have phrased your questions wrongly. If you say to me 'Do you use make-up?' I can say 'Yes' or 'No' and retire into silence once more, leaving you to think up the next move. But if you say 'What do you think of nurses using make-up?' I can't get out of it so easily, and no matter what I say in answer, you have a lead for your next remark. Practise asking questions in this way.

If an argument develops don't try to stop it. Let them work it out between them and lend your support to either side to keep the discussion going. You can put your own point of view in the form of questions, 'Does anyone think these people should do . . .?' or 'I wonder what would happen if the government said . . .?' but once you start saying 'Well, *I* think the unions should be . . .', you have taken sides and you have weakened your power to promote discussion. You may have an interesting talk with one or two of the more articulate patients, but the rest will tend to listen instead of joining in. By becoming involved yourself you have reduced your ability to help the rest of the group.

There are many kinds of groups. Those led by charge nurse or the doctor may be for the purpose of helping patients to solve their emotional problems, but this is not your purpose. In the kind of group described above what is discussed, and even the opinions expressed, are of secondary importance to the fact that you are helping the patients to make ordinary social contacts with each other, to come out from the self-absorbed world of mental illness into the give and take of ordinary life again.

COURTESY

Ordinary, simple courtesy, of the kind you would use among your own friends and neighbours, is a valuable tool in psychiatric nursing. It emphasizes the patient's value as an individual. It shows that you respect him and recognize that he has the same rights as yourself. It oils the wheels of daily routine and lends a personal touch to everyday affairs. The way in which you can use it most effectively is often when you are talking with patients.

Speak to patients as you would to any adult of the same standing as yourself. People do not become un-intelligent, or lose all their knowledge and skill, simply because they have a mental illness. Certainly they may say things which puzzle you and they may behave in a strange way, but this is no reason for speaking to them as if they were children, or to belittle them by calling them all, indiscriminately, 'Dear' or 'Pop' or 'Ma'.

Don't laugh at a patient's symptoms unless you are sure that he thinks they are funny too. After all, you wouldn't make fun of a friend's stomach operation unless you knew that he would appreciate the joke.

Don't discuss patients, in their hearing, as if they were not there. 'Yes, he always sits there. It's hard enough to get him to the table for meals, let alone get him outside, but we manage to take him for a walk sometimes—when there's enough staff on. Of course, dressing him is a headache,' and so on, all with the two nurses standing beside the patient and looking at him from time to time, for all the world as if he were a particularly dim-witted seal in a circus, rather than a human being. Nurses who do this do not intend any deliberate unkindness. They have just forgotten that the patient *is* still a human being, with feelings like their own, although at the moment severely handicapped by his illness.

When you are with a group of patients observe the same rules of courtesy as you would outside the hospital. If you are called away suddenly, excuse yourself to the group, don't just get up and walk away. If someone comes to talk to you about something which does not concern the group, don't stand talking in undertones to each other while they wait for you to finish. Make a brief apology to the group and move out of earshot, so that they can go on talking. In the same way, when you have to interrupt a nurse who is talking with a patient, don't ignore the patient. Say 'I'm sorry to interrupt, Mr E, but I've got a message for Nurse Smith,' or whatever is appropriate.

Finally, having worked hard to build up a good relationship with the patients, and encouraged them to think they can trust you, don't throw it all back in their faces by walking in one morning and saying, 'Well! This is the last time I'll be helping with breakfast in this ward—I'm off to the admission unit tomorrow.'

If you decided to move house you wouldn't just pack up and go, without a word to the neighbours. Think what you yourself would say of someone who did just that. The ward is a community and you are part of that community. Tell the patients as soon as you know that you are likely to be moved. Tell them when you will be going on holiday. Give them as much time as possible to get used to the idea, and help them to turn their attention to the nurse who will be taking your place. The relationship between a nurse and the patients in her care can be strong, and if it is thoughtlessly broken they can be set back and their progress delayed.

True courtesy is simply consideration for other people's feelings and this is one of the principles of psychiatric nursing.

YOUR OWN FEELINGS

As you go from ward to ward you will find that patients behave towards you in many different ways. They may be clinging and dependent, rebellious or aggressive, admiring, affectionate, suspicious or angry. They may want to please you at one moment, and at another stage in their illness do all that they can to provoke you.

It is natural that you should feel irritated by some of them, afraid of others, upset when someone is bitingly sarcastic, or pleased and encouraged when another says he owes his recovery to you. Other nurses feel like this too. So do the doctors and the rest of the ward team.

You need to let patients cling to you without yourself clinging to them. Be a friend to all patients, without seeking their friendship in return. Be prepared for patients to test you out, and when they do, try not to hit back or lose your temper. The place to lose your temper and say just how you feel about it all is in the staff meetings.

Your feelings are just as important as the patients' feelings. Don't keep them to yourself. Talk it over with the rest of the team and be guided by more experienced people. If you do so you will learn how to achieve a consistent relationship with patients—neither so remote that you cannot influence them, nor so involved that you become dependent on them. In this way you will be able to use your own personality to the full, and this is the most valuable equipment you can bring to the service of the patients.

17

Physical treatments for mental illness

ELECTRO-CONVULSIVE THERAPY

If a small electric current is passed through a patient's brain he will have a fit similar to a major epileptic fit. Producing a fit in this way is called electro-convulsive therapy, or ECT. (Sometimes the term electroplexy is used instead of ECT.)

ECT has been found to be useful in helping some depressed patients. If the patient's depression is involutional the effect of ECT can be dramatic and it is for this kind of illness that the treatment is most frequently used. ECT can sometimes be helpful for patients suffering from mania, or catatonic schizophrenia, and it can also be used for those who are actively suicidal, even if their depression is not of the involutional kind. Not all kinds of depression respond to this treatment, but many do and it is used for many patients.

The patient is given an anaesthetic and feels nothing, but after the treatment he is confused and has difficulty in remembering what has happened to him. Although this loss of memory clears up after a few hours it is disturbing for the patient while it lasts.

When the doctor decides that ECT would help the patient he first of all discusses the treatment with him and his relatives, explaining what will be done and what it is hoped the result will be. As the patient will be given an anaesthetic the doctor gets his written consent to the treatment, or the consent of his relative. He then gives the patient a thorough physical examination. ECT is safe and can be given to quite elderly people, but occasionally the doctor may wish to postpone the treatment until the patient's physical condition has improved.

A course of ECT usually consists of one treatment a week for six to eight weeks. For some patients two or more treatments may be necessary in the first week and the course is sometimes extended beyond the eighth week.

Preparing the patient for ECT

The ECT machine can be brought to the ward and the treatment given to the patient in his own bed, but it is more usual for patients to come from various wards to a central unit where three or four rooms are set aside for the purpose of giving ECT.

Patients must have nothing to eat or drink for six hours before the time of their appointment. A person under an anaesthetic will sometimes vomit, and if his stomach is full some of its contents may be sucked into his lungs. This can kill him. As ECT is generally given in the morning this means no breakfast and nothing during the mid-morning break.

Half an hour before the appointment the patient may be given an injection of atropine to reduce the secretions in his lungs. This lessens the risk of respiratory complications when he is recovering from the anaesthetic.

All patients should remove their dentures and leave them in a safe place in the ward. Men should take their neck ties off and loosen their trouser belts. Women should loosen their corsets and remove all hair grips, slides, head bands, hairpins, or anything else they may have on their heads.

Immediately before leaving the ward patients should go

to the lavatory so that they are not incontinent during the fit.

The nurse then takes them to the waiting-room and stays with them until they are called into the treatment-room. Waiting for ECT is worse than waiting to see the dentist and you should keep the patients chatting as light-heartedly as possible until they go in. One of the popular daily newspapers may help, so take a copy along with you.

Assisting with the giving of ECT

As a rule there are two doctors present in the treatment room, one of whom is an anaesthetist. The ECT machine and all other equipment is hidden behind a screen. When the patient comes in all he sees is a trolley on which he is asked to lie down. The nurse makes him comfortable and places a small pillow under his head.

The anaesthetist then gives him an injection of Pentothal (thiopentone) or a similar anaesthetic, followed by a muscle relaxant such as Scoline (suxamethonium chloride).

The muscle relaxant paralyses the patient's muscles so that when the fit takes place there will be no convulsion and therefore no risk of fractures. The relaxant paralyses all his muscles, including those used for breathing. This means that for a minute or two he will not be able to breathe.

To find that you are unable to breathe and that you cannot move a single muscle is a terrifying experience. For this reason the anaesthetic is always given first and the patient is then quite unaware that he is paralysed. Sometimes the atropine is given at the same time as the anaesthetic.

When the patient is unconscious he is wheeled over to the ECT machine. This is a black box, about the size of a record player. Attached to it is a head-band, with electrodes which may be covered with gauze or lint soaked in hypertonic saline.

The nurse checks that clothing is loose at waist and neck, that dentures have been taken out and that all hair ornaments have been removed. This is necessary because tight clothing can interfere with the patient's breathing, dentures can sometimes choke an unconscious patient and pieces of metal in the hair may deflect the electric current and prevent a fit.

She then wipes his temples with a swab dipped in normal saline so that the electrodes will make good contact with his skin, and places a gag between his teeth. Holding his jaw firmly with one hand she takes the headband in her other hand and places it so that the two electrodes are pressed closely against his temples.

The doctor checks that all is ready and presses the switch on the ECT box. The fit takes place immediately, but because the patients' muscles are paralysed all that is seen is a twitching of his face, arms and legs.

The nurse removes the head-band. The anaesthetist takes the gag out and puts in an airway. He then inflates the patient's lungs by means of a breathing bag. This is a rubber bag attached to a face mask. He places the mask over the patient's nose and mouth so that it fits tightly and forces air in and out of his lungs by squeezing the bag. This is necessary because the patient's breathing muscles are still paralysed. Some doctors like to give oxygen and for this purpose the bag can be connected to an oxygen cylinder. The muscle relaxant wears off in a few minutes.

When the patient is breathing normally he is wheeled into the recovery room, with his airway still in position.

In the recovery room

ECT is a safe treatment. Complications are rare, but if they do occur it is far more likely to be during the recovery period than during the induction of a fit.

The recovery room is never left without a nurse while patients are in the room.

Equipment for caring for an anaesthetized patient

should be at hand and the recovery-room nurse should satisfy herself that everything is in order before the first patient is wheeled in.

When the patient is lifted from the trolley on to the bed turn his head to one side, see that his airway is still in place and that he is breathing easily and cover him with a blanket.

Although complications are rare the one most likely to occur is vomiting.

If you suspect that the patient is about to vomit don't wait to make sure. Call the doctor at once.

Similarly, if he is restless, sweating, excessively hot or cold, or seems to be in any way distressed, inform the doctor straight away.

When the patient becomes conscious he will wake briefly, push his airway out and then turn over and go to sleep.

If possible let him sleep until he wakes naturally. When he wakes of his own accord let him sit up and have a cup of tea or coffee and a biscuit, then help him to straighten his clothes and hair before you return with him to the ward.

Sometimes patients are encouraged to get up and go back to the ward as soon as they recover from the anaesthetic. This is poor nursing because it is at this time that they suffer most from confusion and loss of memory. Moreover, other patients seeing them return to the ward in a distressed state may themselves become alarmed and upset. If patients are allowed to sleep through this first period of acute confusion they will be less disturbed when they finally join the others.

Back in the ward

Loss of memory following ECT varies from one patient to another and so does their reaction to reassurance from the nurses. In some the loss is slight and memory quickly returns to normal. Others, although confused, are comforted when the nurse tells them that they will gradually remember. But some will be distressed for the rest of the day and unable to recall what the nurse has said for more than a few minutes at a time.

These patients follow nurses and other patients around, pathetically trying to get their bearings, 'Where am I?', 'What day is it?', 'I can't find my things!', 'What am I supposed to be doing, Nurse?'

The same question repeated over and over again can be irritating and you will feel like getting out of the patient's way so that he cannot bother you any more. You will be tempted to say 'Mr Brown! I told you only two minutes ago!' Try not to do this. Remember that Mr Brown simply does not know that he has asked the same question five times already. Each time is the first time for him.

To have a gap in one's memory is a most disturbing experience and one that is hard to imagine, but most of us have awakened at some time in a strange room, perhaps on holiday or in the Staff Residence, and for a moment have been unable to place where we were, what day it was, or even who we were. For a second panic sweeps up behind us. It retreats at once, of course, but it can give us some insight into what the patient is feeling.

Answer each question simply and plainly. Tell the patient that he has had ECT, that his loss of memory is normal and that he will soon be able to recall what has happened. Try to get him to do something with one of the other patients. A game of cards or draughts will help by fixing his attention on something outside himself. If you can put him with a patient who has had a course of ECT and appreciates how he is feeling this will also help him. Repeat the names of other patients and other nurses when talking to him. This will prompt his memory.

Try to anticipate what he may be needing at any

moment. For instance he will probably forget which is his place at meal times. Take him to his table and make some remark which brings in the names of the patients on either side of him.

Patients who have had ECT need special care for the rest of the day. Apart from the fact that they are depressed, and are under close observation in any case for that reason, there is the additional factor that owing to their loss of memory they may wander away from the ward, or take other patients' things. Nurses should arrange among themselves that one of them is always with these patients until they have fully recovered.

Electro-convulsive therapy is a simple, safe and painless treatment, which has excellent results when given to carefully selected patients. Nevertheless patients are often frightened at the thought of electricity being used on them and the idea of being made to have a fit is repugnant. Perhaps one of the questions most often asked by patients who have lost their memory following ECT is 'When am I going to have my treatment, Nurse?' Their delight when it finally dawns on them that they have already been given their ECT for that day is a poignant demonstration of how much they feared it.

If the doctor thinks it advisable that a patient should have ECT he will discuss it with him and with his relatives, but frequently the patient will come to the nurse afterwards with more questions. Usually he is looking for confirmation of what the doctor has already told him but sometimes he may be worried over a point he has not discussed with the doctor.

It is important that nurses and doctors give the patient the same information. If the doctor says one thing and you say another the patient will feel that he is not being given the truth. He will fear that something is being hidden from him.

The more you know about ECT and the more experience you have with patients having ECT the better you will be able to answer their questions. But when a patient asks you questions about any kind of treatment he is to have, whether it is ECT, occupational therapy, psychotherapy, work in a hospital department, joining a patient's group, or anything else, it is always best to ask him what the doctor told him. This will often help the patient to put his fears more clearly and you are then in a better position to help him.

For instance, when a patient says 'Nurse, what do you think of ECT?' if you tell him it is a splendid treatment and he has nothing to worry about because the doctor will give him an anaesthetic you will not be helping him at all if in fact he has a horror of anaesthetics, as many people have. If, however, you say 'What did doctor tell you about it?' you may learn that although the doctor told him the anaesthetic was quite pleasant he still dreads the sensation of losing consciousness. Perhaps the doctor did not mention that the anaesthetic is given by injection and the patient may be dreading the old-fashioned face mask which he remembers from having his tonsils out as a child. With this information you will be able to reassure him that modern anaesthetics are indeed quite pleasant, with none of the frightening sensations associated with the out-of-date methods.

Most patients' fears of ECT are centred on whether it really is painless and how long the loss of memory lasts. If you approach their questions in the way outlined above you will generally be able to reassure them, but reassurance offered before you know what is really troubling the patient may do more harm than good. Apart from the danger of seeming to give contradictory information you may well give the impression of being insincere and superficial, of having no time to bother with his problems. As a result he may withdraw into himself and lose confidence in you.

You will often notice a marked change in depressed patients who are receiving ECT. Patients who refused food and hardly spoke a word, who wanted to kill themselves and walked about the ward wringing their hands in despair, now begin to notice other people, to enjoy their food and to take part in the life of the ward.

It is important that the doctor should have accurate information about these changes to help him decide how much ECT the patient needs. Nurses should write notes on these patients at least twice a week and more frequently if further progress is noticed. At the same time they should take full advantage of the patient's increased energy to interest him in things outside himself and to improve his physical health.

Patients who are thinking of killing themselves will need special care during the first few weeks of ECT. Often the one thing that has prevented them from committing suicide so far has been lack of energy. They simply haven't had the strength to kill themselves. Now, under ECT, the first change may be increased energy— enough to put their plans into practice.

The nurse should always be aware of this and be more than ever observant of these patients until, with further ECT, their depression lifts and the doctor says the danger of suicide is past.

MODIFIED INSULIN THERAPY

Occasionally the doctor will order modified insulin therapy for a patient.

The purpose of this treatment is to relax him and to increase his appetite so that he begins to put on weight. It is sometimes helpful to patients who are anxious and underweight and who are not responding well to psychotherapy. Patients suffering from drug addiction may also benefit from it.

An injection of insulin is given each morning of the week, except Sunday. Three hours after the injection the patient has a glucose drink, followed by breakfast. He then joins in the ordinary ward activities for the rest of the day.

The amount of insulin needed varies from one patient to the other, so the doctor usually orders 10 units for the first day and increases it daily until he gets the result he wants.

Preparing the patient

The doctor will explain the treatment to the patient and his relatives, telling them how he thinks it will benefit the patient. The kind of patient for whom modified insulin is suitable generally feels that he needs 'building up', so as a rule he accepts the doctor's advice readily and looks forward to having the treatment.

The patient is nursed in bed. He should go to the lavatory first thing in the morning, but he should not wash or have anything to eat or drink. His bed must be in a quiet part of the ward so that he can rest undisturbed by the other patients getting dressed and going to breakfast. The curtains should be drawn so that he is in semi-darkness, and he should be as comfortable as you can make him. If he wears dentures he should take these out and put them in a safe place.

Giving the treatment

The injection of insulin is given at 7 a.m.

The patient's pulse rate is taken and recorded every half hour. Gradually he becomes drowsy, starts to sweat and his pulse rate increases. Each time she records his pulse rate the nurse also makes a note of how much he is sweating and whether he is awake, drowsy, or sleeping.

At 10 a.m. he is given a glass of fruit juice in which 2 ounces of glucose have been dissolved. This stops the action of the insulin.

The patient becomes alert, stops sweating and his pulse rate returns to normal.

Throughout the treatment the nurse should watch the

patient carefully. If she sees any twitching of his face, any tremors in his arms and legs, or notices any restlessness, she should give him the glucose drink at once, although the time may be earlier than 10 a.m.

If the patient has any difficulty in swallowing call charge nurse. On no account should you try to force the patient to drink as the liquid could enter his lungs and choke him.

Complications with modified insulin are rare, but if the nurse is unobservant, it is possible for a patient to sink into a light coma. This is a state of unconsciousness from which he cannot be roused by speaking to him or by touching him. In this condition he is unable to drink and the doctor will stop the action of the insulin by giving glucose either by the nasal route through an oesophageal tube, or by intravenous injection. For this reason the equipment for nasal feeding and intravenous injection must always be at hand when a patient is having modified insulin therapy, but with good nursing it should never be necessary to use it.

When the patient has taken his glucose and is alert again he should be helped to sit up comfortably, with several pillows behind him. The bed should be straightened and the curtains drawn back.

He should then be given a breakfast in which there is plenty of carbohydrate. Carbohydrate is found in foods which contain sugar or starch, such as porridge, cereals, bread, marmalade, jam, syrup or honey and milk. Remember that one purpose of modified insulin therapy is to tempt the patient to eat more. Find out what he particularly likes from this list and do your best to see that he has what he fancies.

See that the tray is attractively laid and make time to sit and chat with him for a while as he eats. Breakfast should be something he looks forward to each day. Your attitude should indicate that the treatment is doing him good and that you are pleased with his progress.

As you talk with him it is quite possible that he will discuss his problems a little more freely than he has been able to do before. You should be ready for this and listen carefully. Report what he says accurately, both to charge nurse and in writing in his Nurses' Notes.

When he has finished breakfast he should have a bath and get dressed. He has his other meals at the usual times with the rest of the patients. Encourage him to have second helpings and let him know that you are pleased to see him enjoying his food. For the rest of the day he should be kept occupied and should be drawn into the general ward activities.

Secondary reactions following modified insulin are rare, but if the patient starts to sweat or feel dizzy he should be given a glucose drink. Some doctors give instructions that patients on modified insulin should be accompanied when they leave the ward and should carry sugar with them, in case they have a reaction.

Half the success of modified insulin therapy depends on giving the patient the feeling that he is receiving special attention from the nursing staff. It is not a treatment which is suitable for all tense and anxious patients, but when the doctor does order it he wants the patient to feel that he is having a good rest, that the treatment is building up his strength and that the staff are concerned to bring him back to full health again, so do all that you can to convey this impression to him in your nursing.

The term 'modified' is used in connection with this type of insulin therapy to distinguish it from insulin coma, a treatment in which massive doses of insulin were given. Insulin coma is not used today.

Two other methods of treatment which were once widely practised, but are rarely used today, are continuous narcosis and prefrontal leucotomy.

CONTINUOUS NARCOSIS

Sometimes patients who are excited, or who are

239

acutely anxious, worried and unable to sleep, will benefit if they can be helped to sleep continuously, night and day, for a short period. This is known as continuous narcosis or sleep treatment, and the aim is to have the patient sleeping for twenty hours out of twenty-four.

The length of the treatment varies. Generally three or four days will be sufficient, but it may be extended to a week or more.

PREFRONTAL LEUCOTOMY

Occasionally you will meet a patient who is so agitated, frightened and tense that life is a daily misery to him. Yet nothing the doctors and nurses can do is of any help. He has had every possible kind of treatment and nothing brings him relief.

Sometimes, after long and detailed consultation with his colleagues, the doctor will advise such a patient to have a brain operation known as prefrontal leucotomy.

This is a drastic operation involving division of the fibres in the frontal lobe of the brain. It is only used as a last resort, and then only in carefully selected patients, but it can sometimes bring about an improvement in the patient's condition when all else has failed.

18

Drugs

When the scientists discovered a new cleansing agent some time ago they called it a detergent. Then some manufacturers took the recipe from the scientists and each produced his own version of a detergent, giving it a proprietary name which belonged to his firm. So we have Surf, Ariel, Daz, which are all detergents but are made by different firms. In the same way, when a scientist discovers a new drug he gives it a name which describes what it is made of. The manufacturer then makes up the scientist's recipe and gives it a proprietary name which shows that it is his particular brand of that recipe.

In this chapter the scientific name will be written first, with a small letter, and the proprietary name with a capital letter, like this—detergent (Surf).

Most of the drugs which are used in the treatment of mental illness can be divided into three large groups as follows:

1. Those which calm people and help them to sleep—sedatives and hypnotics.

2. Those which relieve depression—antidepressive drugs.

3. Those which reduce hallucinations and delusions or reduce tension without making people sleepy—the tranquillizers.

SEDATIVES AND HYPNOTICS

Sedatives are drugs which calm people. Hypnotics send them to sleep. Often a small dose of a drug will act as a sedative while a larger dose will send a patient to sleep, so no hard and fast line can be drawn between these two.

Some of the most frequently used sedative drugs are the barbiturates. Some of these are quick-acting, while others take a little longer.

Examples of the two types are sodium amylobarbitone (Sodium Amytal) 100 mg–400 mg and butobarbitone (Soneryl) 100 mg–200 mg.

Although barbiturates are useful to calm people they can be dangerous if given in large doses over a long period of time because they are toxic. That is to say, they gradually poison the patient. So they are not used as hypnotics.

A drug which is often used to help people to sleep is chloral hydrate. Dichloralphenazone (Welldorm) 650 mg–1300 mg, nitrazepam (Mogadon) 5 mg–10 mg, and flurazepam hydrochloride (Dalmane) 15 mg–30 mg are also preparations which have fewer side-effects than the barbiturates and are used to induce sleep.

ANTIDEPRESSIVE DRUGS

While ECT is used for severe depressions, drugs are often given to relieve milder attacks.

Some of these drugs have a special chemical action on the brain which is not yet fully understood, but which seems to relieve depression. They are called monoamine oxidase inhibitors, and phenelzine (Nardil) 30 mg–60 mg, is an example of this group. Patients taking monoamine oxidase inhibitors must not eat cheese, beans or yeast products such as Marmite or Bovril, nor may they drink alcohol. It is also dangerous to combine these drugs with some others and for this reason the patient is given a card stating that he is being treated with monoamine oxidase inhibitors. He is told to carry the card with him always and to show it to any other doctor who may treat him and to his dentist.

A drug which does not come under this heading but has become well established for its antidepressive qualities is imipramine (Tofranil) 50 mg–150 mg. In action it is more like the tranquillizers. Others are desipramine hydrochloride (Pertofran) 25 mg–150 mg, and trimipramine acid maleate (Surmontil) 50 mg–100 mg. Surmontil has the advantage of being a long-acting drug.

TRANQUILLIZERS

These are the phenothiazine drugs, the drugs which caused such a revolution in the treatment of chronically disturbed patients. They are particularly useful in the treatment of disturbed psychotic patients because they greatly reduce their delusions and hallucinations. This makes them less excitable and more in touch with their surroundings. As a result it becomes possible to use occupational, social and recreational therapy to help them.

Examples of the major tranquillizers are chlorpromazine (Largactil) 50 mg–400 mg, trifluoperazine (Stelazine) 4 mg–45 mg, perphenazine (Fentazin) 6 mg–40 mg and flupenthixol deconoate (Depixol) which is given by injection. Largactil is sometimes given in much higher doses, up to 1000 mg daily.

Because they are used in large doses, these drugs, particularly Largactil, sometimes have distressing side-effects, among which are the following:

Rash on the face and hands, particularly when exposed to the sun. Patients on Largactil should not be allowed to sit in bright sunlight.

Hypotension. The patient's blood pressure suddenly falls and he may faint.

Jaundice. A few patients are affected in this way, but the jaundice clears when the drug is withdrawn.

Parkinsonism. The drug may affect the patient's nervous system in such a way that he walks about with short, rapid steps, his body leaning slightly forward, his arms bent at the elbows and his fingers making small movements as if he were rolling a pill. Saliva may dribble from his mouth. This condition can be prevented or cured by giving one of the following drugs in conjunction with the phenothiazine: orphenadrine (Disipal) 50 mg–400 mg, benzhexol (Artane) 2 mg–20 mg, benztropine mesylate (Cogentin) 2 mg–4 mg, or procyclidine hydrochloride (Kemadrin) 7·5 mg–60 mg daily.

You should remember that the symptoms of Parkinsonism can arise in two ways. Either the patient has been given large doses of tranquillizers, or he is suffering from a brain disorder, as described in Chapter Twelve. In psychiatric hospitals most of the patients who show signs of Parkinsonism do so because of the drugs they are taking, and the symptoms disappear when the drugs are stopped. When you see people outside hospital in the general community with similar symptoms, they are probably suffering from an organic brain disorder. Unfortunately this latter type of Parkinsonism appears to be on the increase.

Largactil can be given in tablet form, or as a syrup, or by injection. In all its forms it is liable to cause a skin reaction in some people. For this reason nurses should avoid letting the drug touch their skin. Gloves should be worn when preparing and giving the injection.

A long-acting phenothiazine, of great use in the treatment of patients suffering from schizophrenia who have been discharged from hospital but still need medicine, is fluphenazine deconoate (Modecate). It is given by injection every few weeks, at the outpatient clinic, the amount and the frequency being adjusted to suit each patient individually. One injection lasts until the patient's next appointment.

Examples of minor tranquillizers, useful in allaying anxiety and tension, are diazepam (Valium) 4 mg–40 mg, chlordiazepoxide (Librium) 10 mg–40 mg, thioridazine (Melleril) 30 mg–100 mg, and haloperidol (Serenace) 3 mg–9 mg daily.

THE USE OF DRUGS

Drugs do not cure mental illness. They can often be a help in the patient's treatment and they can sometimes be a hindrance.

If a patient is so excited and out of touch with this world that it is impossible to hold a conversation with him it will be a great help if he can be given a drug which calms him sufficiently for the doctors and nurses to talk with him. On the other hand if the doctor wants a group of tense and anxious patients to discuss their phobias he will not start by giving them all sedatives so that their fears temporarily vanish into the blue.

Drugs are, at best, a crutch and like a crutch they should be used when not to do so would cause further damage, but they should be put on one side as soon as possible.

GIVING DRUGS TO PATIENTS

The following are some of the points you should think about when giving drugs to the patients.

1. See that the right drug is given to the right patient. When you prepare a drug look at the patient's medicine card and compare it with the bottle or box containing the drug. Make certain that what is written on the

card and what is written on the bottle are the same. If they are not the same ask charge nurse about it.

Secondly, make sure that you are giving it to the right patient. It is easy to mix patient's names when you are new in a ward and there is sometimes more than one Mr Smith. Carry out the procedure laid down in your hospital for the checking and recording of drugs to the letter. Never be persuaded, either by pressure of work or by irresponsible colleagues, to be careless over the checking or the giving of drugs. Because of your professional knowledge the patient is in your hands and he trusts you. You are in honour bound not to abuse his trust.

2. Make sure that the patient takes the drug.

In some wards it is possible to lay a medicine trolley and take it round from patient to patient. In others it is better to take each patient's medicines to him individually. The charge nurse or sister in each ward will instruct you on how she wishes you to give the drugs out.

Most patients will take them willingly, but some may try to spit them out, perhaps because they think that they are being poisoned. Suicidal patients may only pretend to swallow their drugs and in fact will hide them until they have enough to take an overdose.

For these patients it may be helpful to give drugs in liquid form or as syrup. When the patient appears to have swallowed the dose make him talk to you for a moment. It is practically impossible to speak with your mouth full of water without revealing the fact!

Whenever you give medicine to a patient see that he takes it then and there, in front of you. Never let him take it away, no matter how plausible his excuse may be. If you cannot persuade him to take it let charge nurse know.

3. Observe the patient for the effects of the drug.

Every drug is given for a definite purpose, for example, to help the patient to sleep or to lift his depression. The doctor relies on the nurses to give him a detailed and accurate description of the patient's behaviour so that he can adjust the dosage or try another drug, as necessary. Each patient reacts to a drug in an individual way. Sodium Amytal 200 mg may send one patient to sleep, cause another to become excited and have apparently no effect on a third.

Each drug, in addition to its intended effects, also has side effects. Manufacturers try to cut these out as far as possible, but they are always present to some degree. You should be aware of this and report any new symptoms at once.

The following are the most common side effects.

Skin rash	Drowsiness	Dryness of the
Itching	Giddiness	mouth
Jaundice	Palpitations	Tremor
Sweating	Confusion	Facial spasm
		Constipation

DRUG TRIALS

New drugs are constantly being produced and from time to time you will take part in drug trials in your hospital. Some patients will be given a new drug which has just come out, others will have a placebo. A placebo is something which looks and tastes like the drug but in fact has no effect at all on the patient.

Great care will be taken to stop you from knowing which patients are having the real thing and which the fake. Don't be upset about this and think the nurses are not being trusted. As a rule the pharmacist dispensing the drugs is the only person in the hospital who has this knowledge. No doctor or nurse, or any other member of the staff knows how the drugs are allocated. This is essential to the success of the trial.

A good many of us are easily influenced by what other people say and do. I may be going along quite cheerfully when someone stops me and says in a worried voice, 'I say! Are you sure you're all right?' 'Yes, of course. Why do you ask?' 'Only that you look so tired!'

Well, I shrug it off and carry on as usual—and yet now that I come to think of it I *do* feel tired. In fact I must admit I've felt tired all day, only I've just been fighting it off. Better take it easy or I'll make myself ill at this rate. Half an hour later I hear that I've won the ward sweepstake. My tiredness flies out of the window and for the rest of the day I feel full of the joy of life.

In other words, I respond easily to suggestion, and so do many other people. If you know who is having the new drug you may be so keen to observe all its effects that, without meaning to do so, you put ideas into the patient's head. He begins to think that after all he does feel a little brighter today, or maybe he was a bit giddy when he got up this morning.

Not only may you unwittingly suggest symptoms to him but it could be that the extra attention you are giving him is the real cause of his improvement and not the drug at all. It is impossible to make an accurate assessment in this way. Suggestion can only be ruled out if no one knows who is having the drug.

This means, however, that you must observe all the patients even more closely than usual when a drug trial is going on, because nurses' reports carry a lot of weight when the doctors come to judge the value of a new drug.

19

Mental subnormality

Mental subnormality is a state of arrested or incomplete development of the mind, which needs special care or training.

A child may be mentally subnormal for the following reasons:

1. He may inherit the condition from his parents.

2. Something may happen while he is still in his mother's womb which stops his brain from developing any further. For example, if a mother has German measles during the first three months of her pregnancy it is possible that her child will be born mentally subnormal.

3. At the time of his birth injury to the brain may occur from pressure, reduced blood supply or other factors. This will sometimes prevent full development.

4. During his childhood he may have some injury or disease which stops his brain from developing any further, for example a brain injury, a brain tumour, or an infection which causes damage to the brain, such as meningitis.

DIAGNOSIS

The first person to notice that a child is mentally subnormal may be the midwife, who looks after the mother during and immediately following the birth of the baby.

Or it may be the health visitor. A health visitor is a nurse working in the community and one of her duties is to help and advise mothers with children under school age. While doing this she may notice that a child is not developing normally. If, for instance, he is two years old and is still not walking, or if at three years he has not started to speak, she may suspect mental subnormality. On the other hand he may appear normal until he goes to school and it may be the school teacher who first notices his disability.

If mental subnormality is suspected arrangements will be made for the child and his parents to go to an assessment clinic. Here the child will have a thorough examination, both physically and mentally, and if he is found to be mentally subnormal his parents will be given advice and help over his care.

CARE IN THE COMMUNITY

Mentally subnormal children develop best if they can be properly looked after in their own families, and to make this possible the family often needs even more help than the child.

The parents frequently feel, quite wrongly, that it is somehow their fault. They feel guilty and blame themselves or each other. They may give the child so much attention that his brothers and sisters become jealous or even ill as a result. The neighbours may object to their children playing with the mentally subnormal child. The children themselves may call after him, play tricks on him and generally make his life miserable.

The strain on the rest of the family can be enough to break up the marriage or to cause mental illness.

It is important that the child's condition should be recognized early, because then support can be given. The health visitor can support and advise the mother, so can the staff at the maternity and child welfare clinic.

The social worker will keep in touch with the whole family and there are voluntary societies which can offer help of various kinds. At the assessment clinic there are doctors who specialize in the care of mentally subnormal children and they will be ready to give expert help and counselling. There are also a number of parents' associations which have been set up to make it possible for the families of these children to meet each other, talk over their difficulties and exchange ideas. Special care units, which are run like day hospitals, can look after some of the children during the day and so relieve the pressure a little.

Unfortunately all these services are in very short supply. Many parents receive no help at all, and the special care units which do exist cannot possibly deal with the numbers of children needing these facilities.

The area authority is responsible for educating and training the children from the age of five until they are sixteen. A few, who are only slightly backward, can be taught in a special class in an ordinary school. Others will need to go to a school for educationally subnormal children—an ESN school—where the teachers can give them more attention. For the child who cannot benefit from an ESN school there are junior training centres where simple skills are taught.

From the age of sixteen onwards adult training centres prepare the boys and girls for work in the community. Provided they are able to live at home or in accommodation where they can have some help and supervision many of them can be employed in unskilled work and lead a fairly satisfactory life outside hospital, but again there are not nearly enough of these training centres in the community.

Some children cannot be looked after at home, either because they need more attention than the parents can give, or because their presence at home is making the parents ill, and because there is no provision for them in the community it becomes necessary to admit them to hospital.

Others leave school and get work in the community but are not stable enough to hold a job or look after themselves for any length of time. They may drift into drunkenness, prostitution or theft, and be sent by the Courts for compulsory treatment in hospital, or they may come as informal patients on the advice of those trying to help them. So that, in practice, many children and young adults are admitted to subnormality hospitals not because they need nursing care, but because there is no suitable place for them in the community.

CARE IN HOSPITAL

There are psychiatric hospitals in each area which specialize in the care of mentally subnormal patients.

These hospitals have, broadly speaking, two goals in view.

1. To treat any physical disability the patient may have and to make him physically as healthy as possible.

2. To educate him to the full extent of his ability, either to live in the community, independently or with help and supervision, or if this is not possible to live as happily as he can in the hospital.

Mentally subnormal patients can be divided into two large groups, those who are subnormal and those who are severely subnormal.

Severely subnormal patients are usually admitted during childhood, because they cannot be cared for outside, and many have to stay in hospital all their lives.

Subnormal patients are more often admitted when they are in their teens or early adult life, because of unstable behaviour, and many improve sufficiently to go back into the community again.

These two groups are nursed in different parts of the hospital.

252

On admission

Every child is given a thorough clinical examination when he first enters the hospital. Most subnormal patients have reasonably good physical health, but those who are severely subnormal often have many physical disabilities as well. The ear, nose and throat specialist, the dentist, the physiotherapist, the eye specialist, the dietician, the orthopaedic consultant, may all be called in to help. It is particularly important to find out if the child can see and hear normally. Blindness and deafness which is unnoticed can make a normal child appear to be mentally subnormal.

At the same time he will be given a series of tests by the psychologist. These will show how much intelligence he has and will also give information about his personality, for example, whether he is adventurous, confident and aggressive, or shy, inadequate and anxious.

Plan of treatment

When all the results of the examination are known a case conference is usually called to decide on a plan of treatment. Every member of the team has some contribution to make. Nurse, doctor, psychologist, school teacher, occupational therapist, physiotherapist and social worker, all work together to decide what is best for the patient. When the plan is drawn up it will be constantly reviewed and brought up to date as he improves.

Nursing care

Some severely subnormal patients are as helpless as babies. They cannot sit up, feed themselves, or speak and are doubly incontinent. Others may be able to sit up, and like year-old babies can be taken out of their cots to sit in chairs if they are securely strapped in. These children should be cared for apart from the others, in small groups of twelve to fifteen. They need skilled nursing and teaching care and will do so for the rest of their lives. Like babies, if they are to be happy they must have not only physical care but affection too. Most of them are able to respond to the nurses and teachers to some extent and there is usually a warm and loving relationship between them.

Toilet training

For the child who is capable of further development the first aim is to teach him to walk and to go to the lavatory of his own accord. He is slow to learn and constant repetition is necessary, but most mentally subnormal children have sunny dispositions and there is pleasure for nurse and child as progress is made.

Going to school

As soon as he can walk he will go to the hospital school, where the teachers should be specialists in the education of these handicapped children.

First he must use his five senses. He learns, as normal children do, through play, but not nearly so quickly. Coloured bricks, chalks, paints, coloured cards in different shapes and sizes all help him. Gradually he begins to distinguish red from blue, green from yellow. He learns the letters of the alphabet and can count a little. He plays with sand and water, sings and repeats nursery rhymes. Simple ball games help him to control his limbs, so does square dancing or marching to music. If he has difficulty in speaking properly, as many of these children do, he will have special training from the speech therapist at the school. Later he will learn how to tell the time, to read a little, perhaps to write his name, and he may be able to do some form of simple work as he gets older.

The nurses, the occupational therapists and the school teachers work closely together in educating these children and what is taught in the schoolroom is reinforced in the wards, the same methods being used in each case.

Many severely subnormal patients do not develop beyond this stage and the hospital becomes their permanent home. Their parents will be encouraged to visit them as often as they can and to take them out for the day. Some may go out for a weekend, or even a short holiday, depending on their parents' circumstances and resources. For others this will not be possible, but many hospitals have a house on the coast and nurses take the patients in small groups for a holiday by the sea in the summer months. For the rest of the year there are coach rides, picnics, nature study rambles, visits to the cinema, shopping trips and days out in the parks.

Work training

Those who are capable of further development will start training for some form of work.

As in hospitals for the mentally ill the ordinary housework of the hospital can be used to start with and patients learn to sweep and dust, make beds, use a vacuum cleaner and floor polisher, lay tables, serve food and wash up.

Women and girls can learn simple cookery and needlework. There is usually a part of the hospital converted into a flat where they can practise their domestic skills with the help of the occupational therapists and nurses. Some can work in the hospital laundry, the sewing room or the main kitchen. Later it may be possible for them to work outside hospital as maids, cleaners, needlewomen, waitresses, canteen assistants or kitchen hands in hotels, restaurants, cafés, clubs or schools.

Men and boys can work in the grounds of the hospital, and jobs as dustmen, road sweepers, labourers, porters or cleaners may be found for them outside. Many hospitals have an industrial unit where both men and women can learn simple factory work.

If employment can be found for them in the community most patients will start by living in the hospital

255

and going out to work each day, so that they still have the support of the hospital staff when they need it.

Eventually some will be discharged to lead independent lives, but all subnormal people are more dependent on their environment than normal people. If they are insecure, anxious and unhappy they quickly develop behaviour disorders and have to be readmitted for a time. Perhaps the most hopeful situation for them is a residential post with employers who understand their difficulties and are prepared to help them, but unfortunately there are not nearly enough of these. Nor are there sufficient teachers, nurses and therapists in the subnormality hospitals. It has been estimated that more than half the total number of mentally subnormal children in the country, if suitably educated, could later do productive work either in sheltered workshops or in open employment in the community, but in fact many of those children who could benefit are not receiving the education they need, due to the desperate shortage of staff and money in the subnormality hospitals, and to the lack of suitable residential and educational facilities in the community.

Preparation for discharge

While a patient is still in hospital he is given practice in travelling on buses and underground, using money, taking his turn in a queue, ordering a meal for himself in a café, not fighting for everything he wants (as children do), understanding road signs and street notices and all the many things that the rest of us do without thinking about it every day. But in spite of the devoted care of nurses, occupational therapists, teachers and all the other members of the hospital team the transition from hospital to community is a very great step for a mentally subnormal person.

Before he leaves hospital he may have no idea what it is like to sleep in a room by himself, to eat alone or with only two or three people, to work beside someone of the opposite sex, to be surrounded by people who are not in nurses' uniforms, to find his own entertainment every evening and to go home to an empty room.

The strain of this transition is beyond the understanding of the people he will be working with and it is essential that he should have support during the weeks immediately following his discharge. A few hospitals are able to place patients in a hostel when they first go out to work and this is a great help, but there are far too few hostels in existence. The provision of more accommodation of this type for mentally subnormal people is an urgent necessity.

Experiments have shown that when subnormal children are cared for in small family-size units, with a house mother in charge, they make substantially more progress, socially, physically and mentally, than those in hospital. It has been suggested that hospital admissions should be limited to those children who require nursing and medical treatment, and that hostels in the community should be set up on family lines to look after those needing residential care. This would set the grossly overburdened hospital staffs free to concentrate on those children who really need their special skills.

NURSE-PATIENT RELATIONSHIP

Nurses looking after mentally subnormal patients need to be able to create a family atmosphere in the ward. They are acting in many ways as parents and the children will look on them in this light. Most of the children are friendly and eager to please. They become deeply attached to the nurses who care for them, and repay in full measure the affection they receive. A few have aggressive or destructive outbursts which come without warning and for which no cause can be found, but as a rule difficult behaviour only occurs when the children are upset. A good nurse will always be on the watch for anything which could cause jealousy, anxiety or resentment among them, and when they become disturbed she will look first for the cause in the relationships between the nurses and the patients.

Mentally subnormal patients are easily led, some can be exploited sexually and financially if they get into the hands of unscrupulous people and all of them are at the mercy of those with more intellectual ability.

Unfortunately it is only when some tragedy occurs that subnormality hospitals are brought to the attention of the public. Few people know of the devoted care given by overworked staff, often in the most daunting conditions, and the provision of community care for subnormal children and adults falls far short of what is needed, due almost entirely to public ignorance and prejudice.

SOME TYPES OF MENTAL SUBNORMALITY

You may hear the following conditions mentioned in connection with mentally subnormal people:

Down's syndrome (Mongolism)

This is caused by a congenital abnormality in the number of the child's chromosomes. The most obvious features at first glance are the slanting eyes, round head and large protruding tongue. They are all severely subnormal and are generally cheerful, happy, friendly people.

The condition was given the name Mongolism because their slanting eyes and round faces make them look something like the people of Mongolia.

Phenylketonuria

This is the result of an inherited abnormality in the child's metabolism. The condition can be discovered soon after birth by testing the baby's urine and it is thought possible to arrest the mental subnormality by feeding him on a special diet.

European children who have phenylketonuria are always fair haired and blue eyed.

Cretinism

This is caused by an inherited deficiency in the secretion of the thyroid gland. As a result growth of all kinds is stunted, including mental growth. Treatment by giving thyroid extract can bring improvement if started early enough.

Microcephaly

In this condition the child is born with an abnormally tiny head. His face is the normal size but his forehead slopes back almost horizontally and his scalp often lies in wrinkles and folds over his skull. The cause may be an inherited abnormality or it can be the result of his mother having an infectious illness such as German measles during the first three months of her pregnancy.

Hydrocephalus

This is a condition in which the circulation of the fluid in the brain is obstructed, causing the skull to become abnormally large. It can be caused by an inherited abnormality of the nervous system, or it may follow meningitis in childhood. Attempts are being made to relieve the condition by an operation which drains the fluid through a valve.

MENTAL SUBNORMALITY AND MENTAL ILLNESS

A mentally subnormal person may develop a mental illness just like anyone else. In this case he will probably be admitted or transferred to a hospital for mentally ill people. You will also meet patients with epilepsy who are mentally subnormal.

Mental subnormality is quite different from mental illness. In a mentally subnormal person the mind has never developed fully. In a person who is mentally ill the mind has developed normally but has become affected by a mental illness. The following analogy may help.

You and I each have an empty pint milk bottle. You have a pint of milk to pour into your bottle. I have only half a pint. Your bottle is full, but no matter what I do I cannot make my half pint of milk fill my pint bottle. We could say that my bottle illustrates mental subnormality. Now if we forget to take the bottles out of the sun the milk may curdle. It will curdle in the same way in my bottle as it does in yours, although mine is only half full. If you think of the curdling as mental illness it may help you to see the relationship between mental illness and mental subnormality.

20

The patient in the community

When a patient has recovered to the point at which his discharge from hospital becomes a practical possibility the hospital team will have to consider three points.

1. How will he support himself outside hospital.
2. Where will he live.
3. What further help will he need after his discharge.

THE WORK SITUATION

First of all, does he need to earn his own living. If he is elderly and has an adequate pension, or relatives who are prepared to support him this question does not arise. Nor does it if he has an adequate independent income. But for many patients earning their living is the first concern.

Some short-stay patients will be returning to the firm they were working with before they became ill, but for a large number of patients leaving hospital means getting another job. The disablement resettlement officer (DRO) and the industrial therapist know of all the vacancies in the district. They also know which employers are sympathetic towards workers who have had a mental illness and are prepared to help them settle into the job. If the patient sees a post advertised and feels he would like to apply the DRO will be able to say whether this would be a suitable position for him.

The question of whether the patient should tell his

prospective employer that he has been in a psychiatric hospital is one which he and his doctor will talk over together. Generally it is best to do so, but the decision must be made by the patient.

Finding work is very difficult for ex-patients. There is still widespread prejudice against people who have a record of mental illness. Time after time they may be turned down by prospective employers, although they are quite capable of doing the work required, simply because the employer's ignorance makes him afraid of anyone who has been in a mental hospital.

When the patient does start looking for work he will feel encouraged if you show that you are interested. He may want to talk over the sort of questions he is likely to be asked. Women may be anxious about what they should wear and men may need a little tactful smartening up to help them look their best.

LIVING CONDITIONS

Having found work the next question is where will he live.

Many patients who have no home to go to will continue to live in the hospital for some time, going out to work every day. This gives them a chance to get used to normal working again before they leave the security of the hospital. Others will live in a hostel, either attached to the hospital or run by the area authority in the community. Here their meals are provided and they have the company of other people to help them over the initial period of leaving hospital.

One of the great advantages of the hostel is that the patient is not suddenly left to face his new life all alone in a bedsitter. He comes home at night to a group of people whose problems are similar to his own and to a sympathetic staff. They will talk over the day together, console each other, cheer each other up, give each other advice, share information and useful tips, pull each others' legs and generally provide some of the support which is normally found in a family. Meanwhile, if the patient wants to see his doctor this can easily be arranged. The hostel wardens may or may not be trained nurses, but help is always readily available from the hospital when necessary.

Later, when the patient feels ready to do so, he will be encouraged to find himself suitable lodgings in the community.

Some patients will be going back to their own homes. They will already have been home a number of times on weekend leave so they and their relatives will be prepared to some extent for their discharge.

Some will be discharged home, but will attend a day hospital for five days a week. This means that the patient can continue to have treatment, for example ECT or occupational therapy, while his relatives have him at home each night and during the weekend.

The day hospital often acts also as a night hospital and weekend hospital. Patients who are working during the day, but still need treatment which they could not receive in a hostel, can live in the night hospital and have whatever help they need during the evenings and weekends. Unlike the hostel, the night hospital has trained people on its staff and the doctor makes regular visits.

Unfortunately there are not nearly enough hostels and area authorities are slow to provide them, largely because they know that the ratepayers will object to paying for them. Yet discharging patients without giving them adequate accommodation often leads to a situation in which the ex-patient causes trouble and expense to the community that he would not have done had he received the support and guidance he needed in the first place. Without it he may become one of the thousands of vagrant, inadequate, homeless people, who present such a problem, both in time and money, to the social security service, the police force and the area authority.

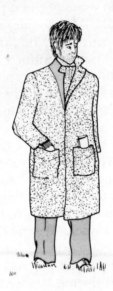

FOLLOW-UP AFTER DISCHARGE

When the patient finally leaves the care of the hospital an appointment is made for him to come and see the doctor at a follow-up clinic in one or two months' time, either at the psychiatric hospital or at the out-patients' department of the local hospital. In this way his progress is watched and further help can be given if necessary. Meanwhile there are several other kinds of after-care available to him.

The area authority social worker will have been told of his discharge. Very likely he will have attended case conferences at the hospital and will have met the patient already. In any case he will be given all the information he needs by the social worker at the hospital. With the patient's permission the area authority social worker will call on him from time to time to see that all is well and to give advice if necessary.

264

The patient in the community

An increasing number of hospitals have an out-patient nursing service. A group of trained nurses visits ex-patients in their homes to give continued support and to report back to the hospital on the patient's needs and progress. Each nurse has her own list of patients and does her rounds regularly—twice a week, once a fortnight, once a month—at whatever interval is best for each patient. Generally the out-patient nurse comes into the ward several times before the patient is discharged. They make each other's acquaintance and are usually on friendly terms before the patient leaves and this relationship is continued, with the patient's permission, when he is at home. This work is highly specialized and the nurses who do it need maturity, psychiatric skill and readily available support from the hospital.

The visits of the social worker or the out-patient nurse can be a great help to relatives who may not be quite sure how they should treat the patient. What do they do when he refuses to take his tablets? Sometimes he stays in bed all day. Should they insist that he gets up? Many of them are too protective. They wait on him hand and foot and are half afraid that he will do something odd at any moment. A nurse, or a social worker who knows the patient can come in and reduce the tension considerably by talking things over with him and his relatives. The firm but kindly attitude of the professional worker gives the relatives confidence and reduces the problem to manageable proportions. They see how the nurse handles the patient and learn from her. Knowing that she will come again next week and that they can get in touch with her at the hospital if they want to, helps them to relax and this, in turn, helps the patient to feel that they trust him.

Some hospitals hold discussion groups for the relatives of ex-patients. Once a month they are invited to meet the doctor and talk over their problems. The doctor helps them to understand the patients' difficulties and gives them advice on what to do. At the same time he learns how patients are getting on. Sadly this kind of help is available to only a few relatives. There are heartbreaking stories of husbands, wives and parents whose relatives are discharged from hospital, who are then left to cope completely unaided, with symptoms which they find frightening and which they do not understand. It is easy to say, 'Go to your G.P.', or 'Ring the hospital for advice', but most G.P.'s have no understanding of and little sympathy for psychiatric illness, while most hospital psychiatrists are at full stretch trying to see the patients still in hospital and have scant time to spare for those who have left. However, where it is possible for these discussion groups to be held they offer an invaluable outlet for relatives' anxieties and so help to reintegrate the discharged patient into society outside the hospital.

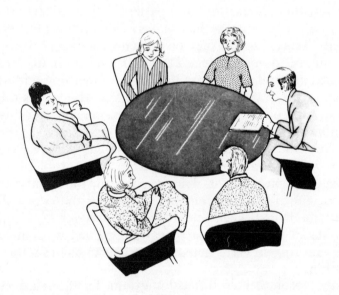

Another useful aid in after-care is the social club for ex-patients and out-patients. This is a club in the community, sometimes run by a voluntary organization such as the League of Friends or the National Association for Mental Health, and sometimes by the hospital or the area authority. It offers social events such as dances, games, debates, and club outings, and is run by the members. Frequent elections are held so that no member can dominate the proceedings for long, and shy ones get many opportunities to take part. Doctors, social workers and nurses are often members, but remain in the background, letting the patients take the major part in deciding policy and organizing activities. There are a large number of these clubs over the country and their number is increasing.

Patients are usually introduced to the club while they are still in the hospital, because they are then more likely to become members when they are discharged. If you are asked to take a patient from your ward to the club, see that he gets to know not only the way from the hospital to the club, but also the way from his home. Find out who are the regular attenders and introduce him to them so that there will always be someone there he knows. Look at the club programme with him and talk about the evenings when he might like to attend. Try to go with him several times before he is discharged so that he begins to feel at home there, and sufficiently confident to go by himself.

THE NURSE AND THE GENERAL PUBLIC

People are gradually becoming less frightened of mental illness, but we still have a long way to go. As a nurse you can have a big effect on other people's attitude—either for good or for ill.

People will try to find out what you think. Friends and neighbours will listen to what you say and take it as gospel truth, because you are a professional person. If you laugh when the conductor says 'Next stop the looney bin!' you have added just that little bit to the ignorance and prejudice which always tries to hold back progress.

No one wants to be forever waving the flag or talking shop, but try whenever you can just to put forward the constructive side. Many people are sympathetic towards mental illness, but they still think patients are dangerous and violent, that you could never trust them again, or that once you have had a mental illness you are no longer quite the same as other people. They still think that doors are locked and windows barred and that nurses carry great bunches of keys around. In your everyday contacts with friends and acquaintances you have an opportunity to correct these misunderstandings and in doing so you do a great service to the patients.

21

Legal matters

INFORMAL PATIENTS

Most of the patients you will meet in a psychiatric hospital have come into the hospital in just the same way that they would come into any other hospital. When they are well enough to leave hospital they are discharged as they would be if they were in a general hospital. There is no legal formality about going into hospital or going out again, so these patients are called informal patients.

DETAINED PATIENTS

A few people need hospital treatment but refuse to take their doctor's advice about coming into hospital. Nothing can be done about this unless the person is a danger to himself or others.

If Mr A thinks the neighbours are trying to harm him by directing an atomic ray at him through the walls he may need treatment in hospital, but if he refuses to come into hospital he cannot be forced to do so. If, however, Mr A becomes so depressed about the atomic ray that he puts his head in the gas oven he has become a danger to himself. On the other hand, if he becomes so angry about it that he takes the bread knife and attacks the neighbours he then becomes a danger to others.

In either of these circumstances he can be compelled

to come into hospital, for his own protection or for the protection of other people.

The Mental Health Act of 1959 lays down the ways in which people may be compulsorily admitted to hospital and the conditions governing their discharge in England and Wales. There are separate Acts for Scotland and Northern Ireland, which differ slightly from the Act for England and Wales.

The Act is divided into Sections. The following are some of the Sections you may hear about in hospital.

ADMISSION TO HOSPITAL

Section 25

The patient can be detained in hospital under this Section for up to twenty-eight days.

The application for admission is made by the patient's nearest relative, or by a social worker. It must be supported by recommendations from two doctors. One of these must be a doctor who is specially appointed by the area health authority for this purpose. The other should be the patient's own general practitioner if possible.

If the patient gets better before the twenty-eight days are up he can be discharged.

If after twenty-eight days he needs more treatment and is by that time willing to remain in hospital, he can become an informal patient.

If he is still not willing to stay in hospital he can be detained for a further period under Section 26.

Section 26

Application is made by his nearest relative or by the social worker, supported by recommendations from two doctors as before, but this time the doctors' statements must contain more detail.

Under this Section the patient may be detained for up to one year.

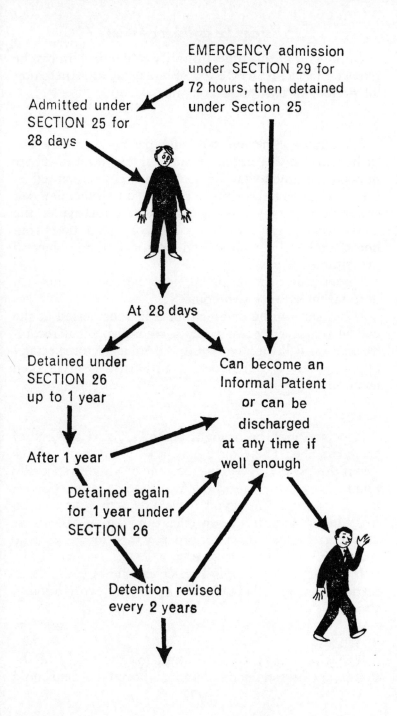

EMERGENCY admission under SECTION 29 for 72 hours, then detained under Section 25

Admitted under SECTION 25 for 28 days

At 28 days

Detained under SECTION 26 up to 1 year

Can become an Informal Patient or can be discharged at any time if well enough

After 1 year

Detained again for 1 year under SECTION 26

Detention revised every 2 years

At the end of this time authority to detain him can be renewed for a further period of one year, and thereafter for periods of two years at a time.

Section 29

Sometimes a person suddenly becomes acutely disturbed and needs urgent admission to hospital. There may not be time to get the doctor specially appointed by the area health authority. In this case an application can either be made by the patient's nearest relative or the social worker, supported by a recommendation from one doctor only, who should be the patient's general practitioner if possible.

Under this Section the patient can be detained in hospital for seventy-two hours.

If he needs to be detained for a further period at the end of the seventy-two hours a second medical recommendation will then be required from a doctor specially appointed by the area health authority. He will then come under Section 25.

Section 60

A person may be brought before a Court accused of some offence. The Court may ask for medical advice about this person. If two doctors, one of whom is specially appointed by the area health authority, think he will benefit more from having psychiatric treatment than from being sent to prison, the Court may take their advice and issue a hospital order, which means that he must stay in hospital for one year.

If necessary the hospital order can be renewed for a further year, and thereafter for periods of two years at a time.

Section 65

The Court may consider that, for the safety of the public, the person detained under a hospital order should not be discharged for a certain fixed period and they may issue what is called a restriction order. The period of restriction is laid down by the Court and may be of any length, from one year to an unlimited time.

Section 72

A man or woman already serving a prison sentence may develop a mental illness and need treatment in a psychiatric hospital. In this case the Home Secretary may order him to be transferred to hospital. This is called a transfer direction. The transfer direction can last for one year. If necessary it can be renewed for a further year, and thereafter for periods of two years at a time.

Section 74

The Home Secretary may consider that, for the safety of the public, the prisoner he sends to hospital on a transfer direction should not be discharged for a fixed period. He may then issue a direction restricting discharge. The period of restriction may vary from one year to an unlimited time.

Section 136

Sometimes a person may start behaving in a disturbed way in the street, or in a shop, or some other public place. It is not always easy at first glance to tell what is the cause of his behaviour. If he appears to be suffering from mental disorder and to be in need of care and control a policeman may take him to a place of safety and he may be detained there for seventy-two hours, while arrangements are being made to look after him.

For example, if Mr A is found weaving his way down the middle of the road cursing to high heaven, he may be drunk, or he may be convinced the atomic ray has got him at last, he may have been taking drugs, or he may be suffering from a brain tumour. Whatever the cause, he is in need of care and control, for his own sake and to protect other people. Someone calls the police and he is taken to what the Act calls a place of safety, which may be a hospital, a nursing home, accommodation provided by the area health authority or the police station.

Special hospitals

A small proportion of detained patients may be dangerous, violent, or criminal in their behaviour. For their own sakes and for the protection of other people they need to be nursed in hospitals from which they cannot escape.

These are called special hospitals and there are three of them for England and Wales—Broadmoor Hospital in Berkshire; Rampton Hospital in Nottinghamshire; and Moss Side Hospital in Liverpool.

DISCHARGE FROM HOSPITAL

Patients detained under the various Sections may be discharged in the following ways.

Section 25
Only by his doctor.

Section 26
1. By his doctor.
2. By written application from his nearest relative.
3. By the mental health review tribunal (see below).

Section 60
1. By his doctor.
2. By the mental health review tribunal.

Section 65
Only by the Home Secretary.

Legal matters

Section 72
1. By his doctor.
2. By the mental health review tribunal.

Section 74
Only by the Home Secretary.

Mental health review tribunals

A mental health review tribunal consists of at least three people, all appointed by the Lord Chancellor. One must be a lawyer, another a doctor and the third a person with special experience in the social services.

Tribunals are appointed for each regional authority and their work is to hear appeals from detained patients.

The patient has to fill in a simple form asking to see the tribunal and the nurses help him to do this if necessary. The three members of the tribunal come to the hospital and the meeting is quite informal. The patient may talk to the tribunal by himself if he wishes. He may also bring his solicitor. Of course, the tribunal will also see the patient's doctor, his nearest relative, and anyone else who may be able to contribute something to help them in reaching a decision.

The tribunal cannot consider appeals from patients detained under restriction orders, Sections 65 and 74. No one but the Home Secretary can discharge these people.

Patients who abscond

Sometimes a detained patient will leave the hospital without his doctor's permission. He is said to be absent without leave, or to have absconded.

When this happens the hospital generally tells the police, the social worker and the patient's nearest relative. An accurate description of what the patient was wearing is, of course, a great help in trying to trace the patient.

If a detained patient manages to live outside the hospi-

275

tal for a certain period without being traced he is considered to be discharged. The length of time he must maintain himself in this way depends on his age and the type of mental disorder from which he is suffering. It varies from twenty-eight days to six months.

Patients who discharge themselves

An informal patient has the right to take his own discharge if he wishes to do so, but this does not mean that you should simply allow a patient to pack his case and walk out because he feels like it.

If a patient with a broken leg in a general hospital climbed out of bed and said he was going home you would tell sister at once and then do your best to explain to the patient how foolish he would be if he did anything of the sort.

The same applies to psychiatric patients and any patient wishing to discharge himself should be persuaded to wait and talk it over with sister and with his doctor before making up his mind. If it is essential that he should remain in hospital and he cannot be persuaded to do so voluntarily, he can be detained for seventy-two hours under Section 30, on the recommendation of his doctor.

The Department of Health and Social Security has issued leaflets setting out the rights of patients detained in hospital, and these are given to the patient and his relatives when he comes in. His doctor also explains to him the conditions under which he is being detained and how he may appeal against detention if he wishes.

DIFFERENCES IN THE ACTS RELATING TO SCOTLAND AND NORTHERN IRELAND

In Scotland

The procedure for the formal admission of a patient is

the same as in England and Wales except that the approval of the Sheriff is also required, whereas in England and Wales the decision to admit a patient is purely a medical matter.

Emergency admissions are made in the same way as in England and Wales except that the order lasts for 7 days, instead of for 72 hours.

In Northern Ireland

A formal admission requires the recommendation of only one doctor, instead of two as in England and Wales, and lasts for 21 days instead of 28 days.

Emergency admissions are dealt with as in Scotland.

Terminology

Patients who, in England and Wales, are said to be 'mentally subnormal' are called 'mentally defective' in Scotland, and in Northern Ireland are described as 'persons requiring special care'.

OTHER MATTERS

Patients on probation

When a Court decides to put an offender on probation it may say that he is to receive psychiatric treatment at the same time, either as an out-patient or an in-patient.

If a patient who is on probation refuses treatment or takes his own discharge his doctor must let the probation officer know at once.

Financial problems

Patients are often worried about money when they are in hospital. In this case the person who can do most to help them is the social worker, and it is essential that nurses and social workers should work closely together.

Patients who receive pensions will go on receiving

them while they are in hospital, although National Insurance pensions will be reduced slightly. National Health Insurance sick pay will be sent to the patient each week until he has come to the end of his entitlement. After that the hospital will give him pocket money. Some hospitals have a welfare officer who looks after patients' money problems and works with the social worker.

Difficulties over the rent and money for the family left at home while the patient is in hospital may be met by help from the Department of Health and Social Security, and there are also various charitable funds available for patients.

Whenever a patient seems to be in any way worried about his money tell sister and she will ask the social worker to come and see him.

Patients' property

All the time a patient is in hospital we encourage him to make his own decisions, look after his personal property and spend his money as he wishes. This is an important part of his treatment. But a patient may own houses and land from which he draws rent, he may run a business, or be in partnership with someone else and have to make decisions affecting other people. It may be one thing to spend pocket money at the hospital shop and quite another to continue to run a business while you are mentally ill.

Many patients are perfectly capable of looking after their business affairs while they are in hospital and, of course, continue to do so. Others may need help in these matters because they are too old or too mentally disordered to do it for themselves. In this case the Court of Protection will act on their behalf.

The Court of Protection is a branch of the High Court of Justice. The Lord Chancellor appoints officers to this Court whose duty is to protect the patient's interests and manage his affairs, under instructions from the Court.

Sometimes a patient who has previously shown good judgement suddenly begins to spend his money recklessly, or gives it away to other people. If you notice this you should let sister know at once, so that the patient may be protected from the consequences of his disordered conduct.

Occasionally you will meet people who are prepared to take advantage of a sick person. If a patient's visitors seem to be trying to persuade him to do something about which he is doubtful, if you hear any mention of buying or selling property, or if you have the slightest reason to think that he is being exploited in any way at all, do not hesitate to go straight to sister.

Making a will

A patient's will is valid if at the time of making it he is 'of sound disposing mind'. This means, if he knows how much money and property he has, can clearly remember his relatives and friends and is capable of judging how much each should have. Questions about wills, or legal documents of any kind, should be referred to sister.

Marriage and divorce

From time to time you will meet patients who are involved in divorce proceedings, or whose marriage partners are thinking of divorcing them.

Although you should refer all questions about marriage and divorce to sister it will help you to understand some of the problems facing the patient and his relatives if you know a little of what the law says on this subject.

A marriage may be annulled if one of the partners was, at the time of the marriage, so mentally ill that he or she did not know what he was doing. It may also be annulled if one partner is subject to recurring episodes of mental illness or epilepsy and the other partner did not know about this at the time of the marriage.

279

Finally, the Court may grant a divorce if one partner has been under care and treatment for mental disorder for a period of five years, whether as an informal patient or under detention.

Offences under the Act

Legal action may be taken against any member of the hospital staff who ill-treats a patient, commits a sexual offence against a patient, or helps a patient to absent himself from the hospital without leave.

Inquests

If a patient dies unexpectedly an inquest is usually held to find out the cause of death and to investigate the circumstances in which death occurred.

Nurses may be asked to attend the inquest if it is thought that they can provide information which may help the coroner. For example, a nurse's observations about the patient's behaviour could be helpful, or her description of what was happening in the ward at the time.

Correspondence

Very occasionally the doctor has to stop a patient's letters from being posted. For example, a patient may write obscene letters to someone. This person may be so distressed by the letters that he asks the doctor not to let the patient post them.

Sometimes a patient will write on the envelope, in place of the address, something which is either quite useless such as a nursery rhyme, or something which is illegible. To post this would only cause a lot of unnecessary work for the Post Office.

The patient's doctor is the only person who is allowed to censor letters in this way and it is rare for him to do so. No nurse may open patient's letters or prevent them from being posted unless told to do so by the patient's

doctor. But if the patient writes to any of the following
people the doctor has no authority to open the letter or
to prevent it from being posted, no matter what he
thinks it may contain:

1. The Prime Minister.
2. The Department of Health and Social Security.
3. Any member of parliament.
4. The mental health review tribunal.
5. The Court of Protection.
6. The patient's solicitor.

In this way the law does everything possible to pre-
serve the patient's right to be heard.

22

The history of psychiatric nursing

Mental disorder is as old as life itself. There are stories in the Bible of people who were affected in this way. Nebuchadnezzar suffered from delusions, Saul and Job had recurring attacks of depression, and Goliath was probably mentally subnormal.

For hundreds of years mentally sick people were thought to be possessed of the devil. Some roamed the country-side as vagrants, others held a position of authority as witches or soothsayers, while every village had its village idiot.

Those who were more violent were imprisoned in large institutions. Many were regarded as criminals, others as clowns or performing animals. Treatment consisted of driving the devils out, or punishing the patient for what was considered to be his criminal behaviour. Whipping, ducking, starving and solitary confinement were common practices and, of course, most patients were chained to the floor or the wall.

On Saturdays and Sundays the institutions were open to the public and for a small charge people could go round and look at the loonies in the cages. It was a popular family outing and just the thing to amuse the children. You could hear the patients screaming from a mile away.

One of the first hospitals for the mentally sick in this

country was Bethlem Royal Hospital, founded in 1247, and the word 'bedlam', which is a corruption of Bethlem, is still used today to describe an appalling uproar.

There were no psychiatric nurses in those days. The patients were guarded by attendants whose main tasks were to administer the whippings and see that the chains held.

This state of affairs went on all over Europe for many years until at the end of the eighteenth century some public spirited people began to press for more humane treatment of the mentally ill. Gradually the public conscience was stirred and the horrifying conditions under which patients were being imprisoned came to light. Doctors slowly became interested in the possibility of medical treatment for mental illness and wealthy businessmen began to give money for this purpose.

In the Bicêtre Hospital in Paris Phillipe Pinel replaced the patients' chains with strait-jackets—still an unthinkable treatment to us today, but a daring experiment for those times and one which will always be remembered. In this country William Tuke founded The Retreat in York, where chains and solitary confinement were forbidden.

The nineteenth century saw a great wave of reform sweep across the country. Many new hospitals were built to house the mentally sick. Most of them were in open country areas, partly to keep patients away from the towns, but also because the doctors genuinely thought that the country air would be good for them. They were asylums, which means places of refuge.

The main treatments were good food, rest, exercise and occupation. Under this kind of régime the attendants found their task was much more that of a nurse than a gaoler. They lived with the patients, often sleeping in the ward. They shared the patients' meals and indeed their lives to a large extent.

As time went on the doctors began to notice that some of the nurses were much more successful than others at preventing destructive behaviour, soothing the noisy patients and rousing those who were apathetic. Dr Connolly, at St Bernard's Hospital in London, began to select his nurses very carefully and suggested that perhaps they would be all the better for some kind of training. Dr Morison at Springfield, also in London, started a series of lectures for his nurses, and so did Dr Browne at Crichton Royal in Dumfries. By 1860 quite a number of doctors were interested in the idea of training for their nurses and they discussed it at meetings of their professional organization, the Royal Medico-Psychological Association (R.M.P.A.—now the College of Psychiatrists). It took a long time to get things moving on a national scale but by the end of the century the R.M.P.A. had set a national standard of training for psychiatric nurses. National examinations were started in 1891 and the R.M.P.A. kept a register of nurses who passed.

It is interesting to recall that it was the doctors who campaigned for nurse training in the psychiatric field, while it was a nurse, Florence Nightingale, who was fighting for nurse training in the general hospitals.

As the years went by physical medicine made great strides. The large voluntary hospitals grew up, with their famous medical schools for teaching young doctors. Inevitably they had a powerful influence on nurse training. The General Nursing Council (G.N.C.) was set up to regulate the training, examination and registration of nurses, and in 1925 it started examining and registering psychiatric nurses.

Gradually the training of psychiatric nurses became more like that of general nurses. Regardless of the fact that 80 per cent of their patients were up and dressed the psychiatric nurses' training concentrated on physical nursing, with psychiatric nursing lagging far behind.

With the coming of the National Health Service the R.M.P.A. examinations were discontinued and all psychiatric nurses were examined by the G.N.C. The

R.M.P.A., however, did not lose its interest in psychiatric nurse training.

During the next ten years public interest in psychiatry grew. Pioneer hospitals began unlocking their doors and allowing patients more freedom. The tranquillizer drugs were discovered and chronic wards took on a positive, hopeful atmosphere. Industrial therapy was introduced, while group and individual psychotherapy became more widespread.

With these developments it became more and more obvious that the psychiatric nurse's training did not fit her for the work she was doing.

The G.N.C. recognized this and began preparing a new scheme of training. The R.M.P.A. pressed for a new training, so did the tutors in the psychiatric hospitals. The World Health Organization set up an expert committee on psychiatric nursing and they too made strong recommendations that the nurse should have a more realistic preparation for the work she had to do. Finally, in 1957, experimental syllabuses of training were introduced which were tailor-made to the needs of the student in psychiatric nursing, and which formed the basis of the syllabuses in use today for student nurses training for registration as mental nurses, or as nurses for the mentally subnormal. But it was not the end of the story!

Back in 1840 Dr Connolly was remarking how much influence his nurses had on the patients. For some nurses they would do anything. The ward was peaceful, the patients occupied and tranquil when certain nurses were on duty, but with others they were disturbed, violent and destructive. Why this should be so he did not know. Today we understand a little more about the importance of the nurse-patient relationship in the treatment of mental disorder. No matter what drugs or physical treatments may be used, the relationship between the patient and the ward team is a vital factor in his recovery and more and more attention is being paid to this.

Some nurses must accept the responsibility of taking charge of a whole ward, of organizing other people's work and of teaching other nurses in the ward. This is the work of the sister or charge nurse and it is for this that student nurses are training. But it has become increasingly clear that we also need nurses who are experts in helping patients, individually and in small groups, through the ordinary activities of daily life in the ward. Nurses who will share the patient's day with him, who will be there when he gets up, who will work and play with him and at the end of the day will watch while he sleeps. Nurses who, because they do not have to take the wide field of responsibility for which the registered nurse is trained, can specialize in the creation of this healing relationship between themselves and individual patients, through the shared life of the ward.

It was the recognition of this need which led the G.N.C. to introduce the enrolled nurses' syllabus in psychiatric nursing, so that with registered nurses and enrolled nurses working together the nursing team should be complete.

23

Looking ahead

Psychiatric nursing is a developing profession and many more nurses will be needed in the future.

As the number of district general hospitals increases more psychiatric units will be opened, calling for more psychiatric nurses to run them. The value of day hospitals is already recognized, and more will probably be built, but they will only be successful if the patient's family receives much more support than is usually the case at the moment. This support can be given by psychiatric nurses working in the community. A number of hospitals already run an out-patient nursing service and many more will probably do so in the future, not only to help the day hospitals, but also to reduce the re-admission rate to psychiatric hospitals. Again, more nurses will be needed to provide this service.

There is a great need for more training and occupational centres for mentally subnormal people, and for more residential hostels and halfway houses for patients when they are discharged from hospital. Most people are even more reluctant to have a hostel in their road than they are to have a day hospital, but pressure is growing. The general public have been made increasingly aware, over the last few years, of the needs of the mentally ill and the mentally handicapped, and area authorities may soon be forced to improve their facilities in this respect.

There may also be an increase in the partnership between hospitals and industrial concerns, with nurses working with groups of patients either in industrial centres outside the hospital or in individual factories, as is done now in some areas.

After a slow start in the 1950s the idea of Health Centres seems to be gaining favour. These centres may include the maternity and child welfare clinic, the school and dental health clinic, the child guidance clinic and the assessment clinic for the area, together with a day hospital, an out-patient nursing service, a patients' club, and a psychiatric out-patient department with rooms for individual and group psychotherapy, social workers, voluntary helpers and marriage guidance counsellors. In this way father, mother and child can be cared for comprehensively, on an out-patient basis.

There will be no real increase in the number of these centres until we can convince people that it is cheaper, as well as thereapeutically more sound, to prevent mental disorder than to attempt to cure it once it is established; but when centres are built there will be a need for psychiatric nurses on the staff.

IN HOSPITAL

In psychiatric hospitals and psychiatric units all over the country, changes are taking place as the recommendations of the Salmon committee on senior nursing staff structure take effect. Other recent developments over the last few years are our entry into the European Economic Community (the Common Market), the Briggs proposals on nurse education, the changes in local government and the reorganization of the National Health Service which came into effect in recent years.

These events have already brought changes to psychiatric nurses and will bring more in the future; changes which will mean renewed hope for many and the opportunity to develop hitherto unrecognized talents, but which to others may bring anxiety and misgivings. New systems of administration, new lines of communication, new clinical and managerial responsibilities mean added stress to some already overburdened staff.

Try to imagine the changes a charge nurse or sister, now in her fifties, has seen since she started her training in the 1930s. At that time custodial care was the common pattern of psychiatric nursing. Nurses did their best to occupy patients, but there were no specific treatments for mental illness. A 'good' nurse was one who could keep the ward quiet, and this often meant heavy sedation and strict discipline.

Then came the discovery of ECT and the development of all the physical treatments—hydrotherapy, malarial therapy, leucotomy, insulin coma therapy. Psychiatric nursing became increasingly physically orientated. The more she resembled a general trained nurse the more approval the psychiatric nurse received. Custodial care was out. The patient must be *nursed*. The nurse must *do* things for him, to bring about his recovery.

No sooner had she become a thoroughly competent physical treatment nurse than the 1950s brought another revolution in the form of the tranquillizer drugs. In a matter of months disturbed, hallucinated patients, who had been in hospital for years, the despair of the nurses and doctors, began to feed themselves, and to answer rationally when someone spoke to them—and without the aid of leucotomy or insulin.

Physical treatments and heavy sedation rapidly declined in favour, and with the improvement in the behaviour of their long-stay patients many hospitals began to unlock wards which had never before been open. This was contrary to all that nurses had been taught for so long, about the need to control patients. Once again they had to unlearn previous training and adjust, not without much heart-searching, to new methods.

Came the 1960s and the therapeutic community appeared on the scene, with its involvement of all staff in the patient's recovery, and its emphasis on the paramount importance of relationships between nurses and patients. No longer could the nurse perform some technical procedure to cure the patient, or administer some drug and leave it at that. She was now called upon to make a personal relationship with him, something she would have been sharply reprimanded for doing when she was a staff nurse in 1940, and something which was in any case difficult enough to achieve, without the added handicap of tradition holding her back.

Small wonder then that some of our senior nurses at times appear to be rather unwilling to change their attitudes. They have lived through so many changes that some of them tend to look on new ideas with rather a sceptical eye.

This is understandable, and indeed the value of tradition lies in its conserving and stabilizing force, which prevents the good being swept away with the bad when change is too rapid. These older people have an immense amount of practical experience behind them, and can offer a great deal to junior staff.

As you go from ward to ward in your training don't make the mistake of thinking that because a ward houses long-stay patients or old people, that there is nothing for you to learn. Some of the most skilled nursing is done in these wards and many of these sisters and charge nurses are specialists in certain aspects of nursing. Each one can teach you something. Find out what it is, and make the most of your opportunity while you are there. It is of little use being able to describe an old woman as suffering from senile and arterio-sclerotic dementia with a depressive overlay, if, after you have bathed her, you leave her in tears wishing she had never been born. Nor does it help much if you can talk brightly about the principles of group dynamics but cannot share your anxieties with your colleagues, or recognize the loneliness behind a hard-boiled attitude. Psychiatric nursing is essentially a warm, human, practical art, and the psychiatric nurse should be an expert in making good relationships, not only with the patients but with her colleagues as well.

There have been sweeping changes in the past and there will certainly be more in the future. A developing profession must be ready to try new methods. So many of us think that the only possible way of doing things is the one we happen to use ourselves. When we do this we are just as full of ignorance and prejudice as those members of the public who try our patience by refusing to have hostels and training centres in their district.

Remember that in 1800 human beings were chained to the floor because they were suffering from mental illness. The people who put the chains on were not monsters, they were ordinary citizens like you and me. They thought they were doing the only possible thing, and when somebody suggested taking the chains off they said he was out of his mind.

To us, looking back, it seems incredible that human beings could have treated one another like this—not in blind rage, but quietly and methodically, day after day, because it was the right thing to do. This is something we should never forget. They were ordinary people like us, and in the twenty-first century ordinary people will perhaps look back on something we are doing to patients today and say, 'How in heaven's name could they have done that!'

With this in front of us we dare not shut our minds to new methods, no matter how revolutionary they may seem, especially not to new methods of treating patients.

This does not mean that we must be foolishly enthusiastic about something simply because it is new, but it does mean that we should be willing to try it out. It means that, as professional people, we must cultivate an inquiring mind, and when we are asked to take part in changes we must do our best to put prejudice on one side.

The methods you are being taught today are the best we know—but they will not always be so. A better way will be found, because there are more discoveries ahead than we ever made in the past. Nurses can either be among the pioneers, or they can hold progress back.

Resolve right now that, when you are faced with something new, before you say, 'They're crazy!' you will first say, 'Let's find out!'.

Index

293

Index

Index

Index

Psychosis, 23, 25
Psychotherapy
  group, 210
  individual, 209
Pupil nurse's role, 286

Recreational therapy, 55 (*see also* Leisure)
Registered nurse's role, 286
Regressed patients, 136
  leisure, 142
  physical care, 136
  relationships, 147
  work, 141
Regression, 4
Rehabilitation, 44
Relatives
  of children, 205
  discussion groups for, 265–6
  of long-stay patients, 148–9, 158
  of old people, 197
Reports
  confidential nature of, 77
  day and night, 76
  nurses' notes, 74
Repression, 5
Restraining patients, 124–5
Restriction orders, 273
Retirement, 20
Rituals, 108
Royal Medico-Psychological Association, 284

Schizophrenia, 27
School, 7
Sex
  in adolescence, 8
  in adult life, 12
Sexual deviation, 179
Sexual disorders, 178
Shaving, 81
Shopping with patients, 145
Sleep, 99, 194
Social clubs, 267
Social relationships, 13
Social therapy, 55 (*see also* Leisure)
Social worker, 33, 40
Special care units, 251
Special hospitals, 274
Staff meetings (*see* Meetings)

Stress
  change of life, 19
  children leaving home, 19
  having children, 18
  in marriage, 18
  old age, 21
  reaction to, 20, 23
  retirement, 20
Student nurse's role, 286
Stupor
  depressive, 114–5
  schizophrenic, 128
Suicidal patients, care of, 118
Suicidal risk following ECT, 236
Suicide, 28
Suspicious patients, 130

Tension, relief of, 220
Therapeutic community, 45
Toilet training of regressed patients, 136–8
Training centres, 251
Transfer directions, 273
Transference, 213
Treatment, 30
  drugs, 241
  physical, 228
Tuke, W., 283

Visitors, 149–50

Walking
  as exercise for patients, 93
  with long-stay patients, 144
  with old people, 191
Ward meetings (*see* Meetings)
Ward reports, 76
Ward team, 49
Washing and shaving, 81
Weekend hospitals, 263
Weight, recording patients', 83
Withdrawal symptoms, 173
Withdrawn patients, 126
Work, 10
  for institutionalized patients, 152
  for long-stay patients, 141, 152
  for mentally sub-normal patients, 255
  for old people, 194
  therapy, 55